ONE IN 88

INFECTING OUR CHILDREN 30 YEARS THE UNTOLD TRUE STORY

RALPH COLON

outskirtspress
DENVER, COLORADO

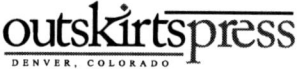

The opinions expressed in this manuscript are solely the opinions of the author and do not represent the opinions or thoughts of the publisher. The author has represented and warranted full ownership and/or legal right to publish all the materials in this book.

One In 88
Infecting Our Children 30 Years/ The Untold True Story
All Rights Reserved.
Copyright © 2012 Ralph Colon
v2.0

Cover Photo © 2012 JupiterImages Corporation. All rights reserved - used with permission.

This book may not be reproduced, transmitted, or stored in whole or in part by any means, including graphic, electronic, or mechanical without the express written consent of the publisher except in the case of brief quotations embodied in critical articles and reviews.

Outskirts Press, Inc.
http://www.outskirtspress.com

ISBN: 978-1-4327-9570-2

Library of Congress Control Number: 2012914619

Outskirts Press and the "OP" logo are trademarks belonging to Outskirts Press, Inc.

PRINTED IN THE UNITED STATES OF AMERICA

Table of Contents

Dedication v

From the Author vii

Acknowledgement ix

One In 88 xi

Introduction xv

Chapter 1   The Bloody Drive 1

Chapter 2   Clinic Of Horrors 4

Chapter 3   The Amoxicillian Experiment 12

Chapter 4   The Final Last Days 18

Chapter 5   The Discharge 24

Chapter 6   The Nightmare Begins Again 31

Chapter 7   Recipe For Autism 37

Chapter 8   Antibiotic Brief 52

Chapter 9   The Amoxicillin Diagnosis 57

Chapter 10   Early Intervention A Must! 67

Chapter 11   My Autism Baby 80

Chapter 12   No Justice For Chris 89

Chapter 13   I'm Sorry For Your Lost 101

Chapter 14 Where Does Autism Come From 111

Chapter 15 History Of Autism 125

Chapter 16 Take Amoxicillin Out 134

Chapter 17 Make No Mistake 151

Chapter 18 Open Your Mind 159

Chapter 19 The Malpractice 165

Chapter 20 Avoid The AAA 171

Chapter 21 Autism Cries For Help 177

Chapter 22 The Autism Rescue 182

Chapter 23 A Law To Remember 184

In Closing 186

Dedication

This book is especially dedicated to my beautiful grandbaby, Chris. Boo-Boo, I call him. He no longer has to suffer great pain, or have the feeling inside as though he was being eaten alive. No more pain. No more tears. No more blood. You are the one, my son, who helped me find the truth behind the lie regarding what they did to you. Every mother, all new mothers-to-be will learn what not to give their baby when the baby's ill, and that they should never put full trust in pediatricians, and most of all, "they will learn why! You stopped my vengeance, my son, but created my revelation. The avenue of justification will suffice. The truth is told. You have saved millions of children from contracting the Autism Affect, and grandpa is so proud of you.

Love You Always My son.,

Daddy Grandpa.

From the Author

The health-related materials of Autism in this book are intended for information and education purposes only. You can rely on this information if you so choose, but you should not rely on this information as a substitute for the advice of your health-care provider, pediatricians and the medical community. Please consult your medical doctors and pediatricians regarding the applicability of my information, as well as of others. The recommendations in this book with respect to any symptoms or medical conditions one may be experiencing at this very moment, is not meant for you to feel any discomfort but for you to be noncompliant.

I am exercising my right of freedom of speech on the subject of my grandson. I consider this important information for parents and new mothers-to-be, with no disrespect to pharmaceutical companies, pediatricians, or medical doctors as they, too, exercise that same right. I have written this book for all parents on a reader friendly basis that they might have a clear understanding of the information herein. It is my desire that parents be able to conclude the truth about a certain drug pediatricians prescribe for our children. I am placing the information in a chronological order that will demonstrate to you a very upsetting conclusion.

After reading this book, we should all be in prayer that our children could receive a more respectful and informative quality of health care—health care that they deserve. This matter must be treated with the utmost concern, as one would be concerned for royalty. New laws should be implemented; pediatricians must allow parents to receive quality information about the drugs they prescribe for our children, not just the side effects they print. They must share the danger levels of each drug, involving 1) our children's immune system, 2) digestive tract, and possible disruption of vital organs within the child if a drug is taken excessively, until the danger levels reaches a period of growth period which results in a disease with no end in sight for the child. Most importantly for pediatricians, they must maintain a record to share with parents of all the cycles their children have experienced of the same drug since birth. Enforce it!

RC. Grand Pa

Acknowledgement

I and millions of parents in America admire the studies from these professionals. The medical community, in my opinion, may or may not have taken these studies serious enough to implement a preventive action for our children by eliminating the source that I believe is harming our children, I will never know their true intentions but assume otherwise. It is fair to say that we have never seen the subject matter enclosed being researched or discussions in the media of possibilities of altering our children's system due to these studies completed some years ago; and I thank these professionals for their passion of care to our children.

Miss. Kelly Dorfman –Co-founder Developmental Delay Registry. Licensed Nutritionist. The Developmental Delay Registry.

Dr. Joan Fallon - Studies with Children and Antibiotics.

Dr. James Lowenstein - Study on Excessive Antibiotics on children.

Dr. Owen Hendley - Study on Bacteria and Antibiotics. Placebo Recipients -Vs- #1 Drug On children.

The World Health Organization - Warnings of Diseases caused by excessive Antibiotics Amoxicillin #1.

The Agency for Healthcare Research and Quality.

Terry A. Rondberg, D.C. - Under the Influence of Modern Medicine.

ONE IN 88

The United States has a very high population of autistic children and adults. One in 88 children is being diagnosed with autism today, the majority of which are diagnosed at three to five years of age after a normal birth. One in 54 boys is diagnosed with Autism today. The growing numbers of children being diagnosed with autism (1 in 10,000 children in the 1980s) traveled faster than a speeding bullet downhill to 1 in 150 children being diagnosed with autism in 2002. In 2006, 1 in 110 children were tagged with autism. Today, 2012, 1 in 88 children are diagnosed with autism.

The population keeps growing year after year, faster than any known disease in children. Many doctors and researchers have put their abilities to the test, but could not conclude what is causing our children the Autism epidemic. In all cases of researchers, they draw their own opinions and assumptions on this escalating autism dilemma with our children, but to no avail. They have no concrete answer. Some have expressed disturbing opinions connecting the topic of vaccines and Autism. Over 60% of parents blame vaccines for causing autism. Some argue the problem is genes or environmental, with no facts but only assumptions and possibilities in every description involving the Autism affect.

However, there is a case where a Judge ruled in favor of a child in a case involving vaccine. This left many top medical doctors and researchers baffled among the medical community. Could this be the case that answers the questions about the relationship between vaccines & Autism? Until this day a majority of professionals argue this is not the case! If that were the case, you and I, and three quarters of our population in America would be Autistic. That decision coming from a judge was not ruling that vaccines cause autism; that decision was based on the ramifications of the case involving one child and the claim of vaccines. It was a technical issue that ruled the judge to make that decision in favor to the child. The sad part about this is that the actions of a few people have convinced many parents in the past even to this day not to vaccinate their children. It is sad to say we are seeing many cases of babies contracting different diseases and even death for not being vaccinated; cases of measles are at record numbers. I believe it is stories like Dr. Wakefield's, Jenny McCarthy's, and others that convince parents not to vaccinate their children. These are respected people of stature and I have no animosity toward them.

It's like a psychological message to the mind after reading their stories and knowing it involves the readers' children not turning autism as the authors describe in their books. Through their writings, the reader will follow the authors' experiences step by step. One can assume after reading someone's experiences involving Autism in this case, we tend to follow the authors' solutions in which they tell us what we should not do, instead of what we should do. I guess in my case, too, you will see that the outcome will be the same.

The only difference between my story and theirs, is that the information in my story is not conjecture. You will be the deciding reader on the subject. The Big Question Is - **Why is this happening to 1 in 88 of children 1 in 88?** Some say there may be other causes for autism - Diet, Body Fat, Candida Overgrowth, Glutathione, Longevity and Quality of Health in Fetal Nutrition. Even though these explanations may seem to make sense, it is not logical or common to see our children developing autism like this at such a fast high rate of production, compared to the children of the 1980s at 1 in 10,000. There has to be another logical answer as to why. In thirty years, the fast growth of Autism among our children must have an explanation. In life, everything has an explanation and you do not have to be a person of stature to have the answer. Compared to past history we can say something is very wrong here!

Dr. Sanja Gupta from CNN confirms the fast growing population of autism has no explanation. Dr. Gupta says everyone is talking genes and environment, but the truth is that it's impossible for the gene affect because the genes in our human body do not change that fast and it would not account for the 78% increase of autism in the past ten years. It would take hundreds of years for one gene to change, unless of course twins are involved. There are some researchers who have voiced their findings and opinion on this problem; they may have found another possible cause for the autism development in children. It is a tragedy that these good researchers and their study stood ignored by the medical community, claims their research needs more evidence on the subject. How much more solid proof do they need?

Well, I have plenty of evidence, and if the medical community had listened to these past studies, we would not have the rise of autism we see today in this country. I would not have a grandchild I love very much suffering with Autism the way he did by four pediatricians and this drug they use on children.. It is my grandbaby's story that has offered evidence to answer the question regarding how hundred of thousands of children are being affected with autism today and why. The Autism Affect that is being introduced to you right here, right now, has been with us for three decades, and we allowed this to happen.

Come with me now and witness for yourselves a story that must be told with an answer to why many children who are born with no problems, a good birth, then turn victims to this terrible disease by a recipe created thirty years ago. This is a thirty-year-old recipe that changes the mental development of our children that we see today. After you see what I see, you will conclude that the facts speak for themselves. You will conclude that the candle may not be lit but the fire is in the candle. The big question for you and me is, was this deliberately planned? On the other hand, is this just an accident spinning out of control, blinding our medical community for years? In the end the parents take the fall and the pharmaceutical companies take the profits. You Decide!

INTRODUCTION

I will tell you about a baby boy who represents the harm that many children are going through today with the development of autism. This represents a harm against our children that goes unnoticed. It is a true story of negligence of a special kind that is being practiced every day throughout pediatric clinics in this country without parents knowing about it. For thirty years it has saved lives, but at what cost?

We never worry about the inner effects destruction it can cause when it comes to our children's anatomy. We don't fret about serious consequences because we trust our doctors. The bloody experience that this baby went through, the pain and suffering was the revelation that I should learn and research for answers. It makes me cry to have learned that this baby is not alone; there are thousands of children who have fallen to this wave altering our children's development without the public recognizing the problem.

This beautiful six-month-old baby was born a normal child, but fell victim to an inner lifeline of infectious deadly bacteria in his system. These spores of bacteria created inside of the baby's system is not passed on by the parents, but by the pediatrician who continued giving the baby the same "cure" using this dangerous drug. For a great many it will damage his or her system, changing their development as time passes without parents realizing it. The damage this baby's system endured, however, goes beyond comprehension.

This little baby's system was shutting down one day at a time until the time limit was up. These bacteria, of course, will either kill him or change him forever. For the millions of babies and toddlers that do survive, then come the effects of autism. The alteration takes affect.

The interference begins in the mind. Their motor skills, then the cognitive skills, social skills—from there a diagnosis of autism between 3 and 5 years of age; and—for the children that slipped between the cracks—between 5 and 10 years old, they also will be diagnosed with Autism. It all could have been prevented thirty years ago before this child was even born. Over the years, there have been children who do not survive the cycles of treatment, and then the parents blame themselves. Of course, my heart goes out to the families and the children of a lost one. Not all children reach that point of no return, landing in hospitals.

However, for the thousands of children that do not land in hospitals under this type of treatment, many are living their lives day by day at home. Their system is changing slowly from the normal development into a delayed development in their minds at a certain period in time. As this recipe of destruction among our children falls into place, time is all that is needed before the development of autism is complete. This is the cause of our mass production of autism today. It has been with us for 30 years, and I am here to show you. People today do not know what is going on with Autism and our children, not because we are uneducated or any other reason you may think of. After all, we trust the news media and our doctors for information, besides developing our own source of information. We trust our pediatricians and the medical community with our children for answers, as we trust in humanity. After everything I have learned, the autism of this beautiful baby boy could have been prevented.

For over thirty years the numbers have sky rocketed with hundreds of thousands of babies who fall victims to this type of suffering and inner system alteration. Why? One thing is clear: we see in the news at many times how our children in America are being over-medicated. Pediatricians' today attempt to assuage our children's pain with medicine which unleashes a feeding frenzy into their system. They know all too well, crossing the limited cycles the children can take in their system would cause harm and developmental problems for the children's mind and future.

This is something that has been ignored for far too long and is time for them to step up to the plate and take the right approach on families with this issue. It is time to look at this problem and try to slow it down or stop it by educating the public on the true preventive measures that exist (aside from all the uncertain possibilities the public have been receiving for years from the medical community). I'm sad to say many pediatricians know about this type of destruction inside a baby's system. What this baby went through has opened my mind to what must be done to stop this from happening to another child—a recipe that is changing our children with no hope of recovery. A recipe is being used against our children, at the same time keeping the parents blind to the effects through manipulation tactics coming from our own pediatricians themselves and winning our parents' confidence that everything is going to be alright! A recipe I call it, because of the length of time—the cycles it takes for the development of the Autism affect to take place.

I sometimes ask myself if I'm wrong about the only logical true evidence left in answering the Autism population question. Would that change anything today? Of course not. Can you hear the laughter? I will just be another person to laugh at in this world of sadness and pain. However, if I am right, we will save millions of children from contracting autism from this un-noticed recipe that harms our children. Moreover, we would just keep living our lives, but only this time looking to our pediatricians for more information on the prescriptions they give our children.

The cycles reach a dangerous level that can produce spoors of bacterium in the baby's system, and records of these cycles must be kept for the patients to have. If indeed I have found something to factually think about, then we have something to go on and parents themselves can finally have some answers as to why and what to watch out for in prevention. I, for one, truly believe the medical community knows why this is happening to our children but refuses to publicize the matter, as we have witnessed for thirty years.

Understand something here; when it comes to finding a cure for your baby's ailment, prescriptions are provided. What you feed into the baby's system for that ailment will affect the baby in a good sense or in a bad sense, and we worry about the outcome. In this case, the government health department has allowed permanent harm to our children for not looking into the matter thirty years ago. Parents are blinded by the performance of the drugs their pediatrician introduces for their children's ailments.

They gain the parents trust by taking away the baby's pain, as if that is all that matters, nothing else. However, is there something else? It's all about wanting to see your child out of pain but not realizing certain important factors may occur in the future for your child depending upon what is prescribed to your baby on a random basis. The danger level of using that drug randomly every time your baby gets sick is adding injury to a permanent developmental problem years later.

These levels of danger that our children have been reaching through time have caused some changes, changes that are not explained by your pediatricians until the time limit is up and the child shows signs of dysfunction. These changes in your baby's system can be explained by your pediatrician; if anything they always refer you to a specialist. After you read this story, you will see what I see, and then you will ask yourselves why?

Many times, we walk into a clinic, and we can see pediatricians are too busy with many patients to pause and educate their patients on the consumption of the deadly drug prescribed to their child. For them, explaining is time consuming. They should be educating patients on how much their child has consumed since birth, and the danger level of alteration using the drug. "It is your responsibility to read up on the medicine and its dangers" - would be their reply to you!

I believe is the responsibility of the pediatrician to educate us on every medicine, and all options available for a safer recovery - not a quick recovery, but a safe recovery—one that will not cause our children any future problems! This beautiful baby boy is my grandson. I love him very much. The suffering, the pain and misery my grandson went through, the suffering my family and me are still going through - no baby and his family should ever have to go through in the so-called great country of ours! He was not born with Autism.

He was born a normal child, playful and jolly through his first six months of life before he fell victim to an inner developmental alteration that was evidenced after the time limit was up. Something was growing inside his body to change his development through an unnoticed process, which has been with us for three decades. He was diagnosed with Autism at 16 months old, after the recipe was fully cooked inside his body to contract developmental problems from this timely manner for the autism to take affect. Of course I would not make this claim without facts. I came to learn of all this and the thirty-year growth of Autism, after they did what they did to my baby's life. It is a shame how many professionals feel the death of one child outweighs the death of many; it made me sick to learn that. With my studies it seems thousands of children die from this incredible recipe of destruction, not only abroad but in our own territory; and our children's defenses are helpless against the concept of greed in this country, blinding them from the outcome our children face.

The news media do tell the public about the children who die each year in our hospitals, due to viruses and bacteria in their systems. With no disrespect to the blind in this world; we are just blind as a society to the reality of the situation; we can't see! The system knows that. Our blindness is well understood, but do we have to stay blind forever? Its time to put on our glasses! Allow me to share the facts, and explain what is really happening to many of our children.

As for me, I believe one child's death is one too many. What I will share with you leads to a shocking conclusion that can put the production of autism in this country to the norm of 1 in 10,000 children from back in the 1980s. It is you, "The People" that can make this happen! We must destroy the source that is affecting our children with autism today. For the children who understandably are born with Autism at birth will hold statistics at the normal level of production. I believe we can help the group of children who are born normal but contract autism in later years (three to five years of age). By getting this story out, we can start the process of slowing down the autism affect. The objections of the source causing this problem started thirty years ago, at the same time Autism started increasing among our children using that same source. I vowed vengeance upon the four pediatricians who destroyed my beautiful little boy's life and future, but that plan in the long run will bring misery and pain to my love ones and to me in the end.

Therefore, my next best weapon turns out to be the pen, which is mightier than the sword. I found the strength to write this story, and hope you understand that what is in front of you could be the answer we all seek to help the future of our children. This story records how blindsided we parents have become, not being able to see our children becoming victims of autism through this process unnoticed.

There are parents who have noticed the Autism Affect on their children through the use of the prescription source, but their concerns and findings stood ignored by the medical community in the 1980s; why? Why did our government in the 1980s allow this to happen to our children? This story will finally wake us up and put an end to the blame game on parents and assumptions. This, of course, is not the parents fault. This shows how vulnerable we are to the medical community and abroad, using our trust, using our compassion and mixing it with their business ethics so they can stay afloat. This is how we good people and families have become, and we must be vigilant in our lives—especially protecting our children. They do this with a systematic system that works, knowing we Americans live on trust and we believe anything they tell us. One of my challenges is that you take a different perspective when dealing with the medical community and your pediatrician concerning your baby, child, or newborn when it comes to your child's medical ailments.

Our children are suffering from the very same person who is in charge of finding a cure for that child - your pediatricians!

One may say, chances are that pediatricians themselves may not realize what they are doing to our children; but I do not buy that. Doctors are always on the path of knowledge when it comes to medical issues and medicine, especially involving children. After a time of pain and sorrow regarding what happened to my grandbaby, I conducted a three-year in-depth research and came across something that has been harming our children for three decades.

The cause is something we all know too well, but never realized how serious it affected our children. We do not care to know simply because of our trust in the doctors who treat our children. Sometimes trust is the cause of our blindness, and then suddenly as time passes we come to realize how wrong we were to trust the pediatrician after the problem occurs. We then blame ourselves with good reason in the end. I believe I will answer the problem of 1 in 88 children being diagnosed with Autism today. And the numbers are growing at an alarming rate day by day. My heart goes out to all the children that are born perfect in the eyes of God, only later to find out that man would alter God's plans.

Now God's children have been compromised forever in their lives. My family and I are a caring family whose lives have been changed forever over our grandbaby's torture, and his new complicated Autistic life. How this occurred is a memory that will live in us forever. It's time for some facts about 1 in 88 children being diagnosed with Autism after a normal birth.

I pray to God that he makes you see what I see during the reading of this book. Is it time for a recovery process to take hold for the future of our children? Our government has yet to offer an answer to the mass production of autism? I am sad to say that indeed our government dept. of health in the 1980s are at great fault here for our children who are born normal, then in later years are diagnosed with Autism. They were at the helm to stop it, and did nothing!

The information in this book is a look at a new beginning to a solution to what has been shown about autism. The explanations we have been receiving from the medical community for years on autism manifesting itself years after a normal birth just do not make sense. I offer first-hand experience, being physically in the presence in the recovery process of one of many children who fell victim to this un-noticed Autism Affect. For me, I feel that these researchers and the medical community are holding something back, and the information is systematically secured. The future outcome for a disrupted immune system in a baby would bring millions to the table. Autism is just one disease of many that continues unabated, so they can keep collecting from the money river. This is how I truly feel about many doctors in our society today; this is how they think. This is the impression they give the parents between the lines. You have to read this book in it's entirely to view the evidence. At times you may read something you read already, but understand it had to be said again. Sometimes my friends it takes repitition to learn and remember important information that will dwell upon in your mind, so when you conversed the subject matter it will come to you at a moments notice so you can recall what you have read and learned, especially when the information is about your children's health and development, and the corruption that exist.

You have to follow the story line, every page has an explanation as to now, why, how, and because. Focus on the subject matter. See for yourselves what it took to change from 1 in 10.000 in the 1980s, to 1 in 150 in recent years and how today, 2012, 1 in 88 children are being diagnosed with Autism. We parents are fighting what seems to be a hopeless war protecting our children. Our babies' and children's future are in danger with no end in sight. You have read Jenny McCarthy and Dr. Wakefield's reasoning, basing Autism on vaccines gone awry.

However, this is something I have always said was far from the truth based on the growing population of autism as we are witnessing today. Vaccines are not the answer.

Now you will read what happened to my baby; then decide who is right - your pediatrician's opinions on the subject, or the reality of what has been going on here for thirty years that is being shared with you in this book. The truth of the growth in Autism discovered in this book has been in front of us for three decades.

We have been redirected by other possible causes explained by professionals for us to see the truth, the real puzzle, the real formula, the real recipe! We are blind because they hold the title to our common sense. You will note the vast climax of the Autism population is taking hold between the 1980s and today, 2012; this thirty-year time span is very important to remember while reading this book.

While some may argue that I should not include the medical community for natural diseases, I say that is far from the truth; I say to all who are reading this book to look at the facts. It's time to stop and listen to your heart and mind when it comes to your baby and you. Think logic! Stop putting all your trust in your doctors, leaving your mind satisfied that everything is going to be O.K. For many this will be a wake-up call today, for the truth has come to focus because of the torture a beautiful little baby boy went through, and a grandfather who demanded answers………….and found them…….and was shocked!

*The following takes place on
Saturday, September 11th, 2005 on a dark*

Rainy night driving on an interstate to St. Petersburg.

1
THE BLOODY DRIVE

Saturday Sept. 11th, 2005. It was a long drive and the blood was pouring out of the baby's diaper. The car seat is full of blood. Blood is coming out of his eyes. My wife is holding the baby, just crying, trying to do everything she can to make it a comfortable ride for the infant. The baby is screaming and crying, blood's all over my wife's clothing. It is late and I know that I have to make a stop somewhere so we can change the bloody diaper.

Every minute counts because the baby is showing signs of death. The smell of death is in the air, like a dead body decomposing. You can actually smell the blood coming from the baby. The blood is in his eyes, coming out from the corner section of his eyes. It is raining very hard, the time is about 11:00 pm, and I know I was nowhere near the hospital. The baby is crying and in so much pain.

I see a late night gas station so we pull in under the gasoline overpass night lamps. The car smells like horror. My wife begins to change the bloody diaper. She quickly puts the diaper in a bag to save it for the doctors at the emergency room. The baby is crying in a weak voice, my wife is crying in pain and I am too. My wife puts two sets of pampers on the baby, as she has been doing since early morning to try to control the blood coming down the baby's legs. The blood is mixed with black acid diarrhea that eats away pampers. Once back in the car I know somehow I have to hurry up and try to reach the highway. I know once I reach the highway, it will be a much easier and faster drive to the hospital.

I tell my wife to make sure all seatbelts are fastened and I drive without stopping at every red light we see. I even drive past cars on the road shoulder and through the intersections. My thought is hoping a police car will stop me, so he can see the emergency and hopefully escort me all the way. If there is an angel protecting me on this journey to the hospital she must have been with us. It is raining hard and I am lucky, because God only knows I should have had an accident the way I am driving. It is taking a long time to get to the highway and I start to pray, crying along the way.

All of the sudden, I am somewhat relieved, but am afraid that my baby is not going to make it being that he is losing so much blood; the highway is in front about ¼ mile down. As I jump onto the highway, I am happy that there is hardly any traffic because of the rain at that time of night. It is easy driving from that point, but my mind is going crazy hearing the screams and cries from my baby and my wife. I can see the pain and suffering my wife is going through in the car through my rear view mirror. Finally, I get to the exit 22 off highway 275. I exit and drive through all the lights. I can feel that the hospital is about two minutes away. My wife is screaming to hurry up, yelling at me. As I turn the corner, it is a welcome sight to see the hospital. I drive straight up to the entrance of the emergency room without parking the car correctly. I grab my baby in my arms, but he stops his crying and just starts to dangle his arms hanging down from mine. I quickly run through the doors of the hospital. Without hesitation, I yell to save my baby's life, and without question, they quickly escort me through some doors. I can see the emergency room doctors approaching me and grabbing the baby off my hands.

It seems that these emergency room doctors were waiting for us. I did call them before I left my home to explain my emergency, that's when they gave me an order on the phone to bring the baby to the emergency room ASAP. My wife followed the baby with the doctors to the back of the emergency room. I then gave them my baby's information, age, insurance and the reason my baby was in that condition. After the registration, a representative of Department Children and Family Services asked me questions.

I thought the worst when they started to ask me questions about my baby's dying condition. After I told them everything about what had happened to our baby, I had them in tears. They could not believe my story but knew that it was true. Then they let me go and I could feel their sorrow for our baby. I asked them, "How about the people that did this to my baby—are you going after them?" They told me no, that their job is only the children. I could see it in their eyes - they felt bad in telling me that. I was in shock to hear this. They said to me – "Good luck."

As I walked over to the waiting room, I could see my wife was just crying and I sat next to her with a hug. I could not believe what I just heard. At that moment, I just started to think in my mind how my baby landed in this emergency room almost dead at 15 ½ months old, and would he survive?

As I'm sitting there in the emergency room crying with my wife I start to think back, way-back, when I first met four pediatricians who destroyed my baby nine months before my baby landing here in the emergency; Just remembering that first day I stepped into their clinic ………It all came to my mind at that moment, a journey back in time to the beginning………Just remembering how and why………..

2
CLINIC OF HORRORS

<u>December / 2004</u>. We've had our grandson four months now. He is growing playful and full of life. He is our joy. His birthday was sad. He was sick, had a cold and a fever that day. The weather here in Florida for December was not freezing but it was a little chilly you might say. Therefore, on his six-month birthday he had to spend it inside a nearby clinic.

On that day, we met Dr. Marlene and she examined my grandbaby and gave me two prescriptions, one for his coughing: CARBAXEFED DM and one for his fever: IBUPROFEN 100 /5 ML SUS for 14 days. I thanked the doctor for treating my baby. She was so nice and professional. I felt a little rusty; after all, it had been many years since I last walked into a pediatrician's clinic.

The next evening I noticed that the baby started to grab his ears; it looked like he was in pain. December 10th I took the baby back to the clinic and my baby was seen by another doctor, Dr. Marlin. Dr. Marlin checked my grandson's ears and found the beginnings of an ear infection. He also found a little wheezing sound coming from the baby's chest. I was puzzled because two days before the other doctor did not say these things to me, but I just brushed it off. The doctor explained to me that the baby may need ear tubes later on, but first he was going to try mild antibiotics to kill the infection. He prescribed for the ear infection **Amoxicillin 200 milligrams** for 10 days. I did not know much about antibiotics or much of anything when it came to medicine. I was a grandfather and my day of rearing babies was over but I knew I was not going to let that stop us from rearing our grandchildren.

I was confused because I went to the clinic two days earlier for a cold and a fever and now the baby has an ear infection. He said the most important medicine for killing the infection is the Amoxicillin. I had my full trust in the doctor, so I did not worry much about anything. My heart started to go down in sorrow that my baby had this ear infection on top of everything else.

Dec. 21<u>st</u> - Within the two weeks of giving him Amoxicillin, it seems that the ear infection started to subside and I was relieved somewhat, but his coughing had gotten worse, and all of a sudden, he had a very bad breathing problem that was very noticeable. I did not like what I saw and I knew it had to be the medicine. I gave him some more of the cough medicine I had received weeks earlier.

January 18, 2005 - Even though the ear infection last month looked like it went away, all of a sudden, the ear infection came back and the baby was crying loudly. I ran out of the medicines so I had to go back to the clinic. I went back to the clinic and told Dr. Marlin that my child's ear infection came back, and his coughing and wheezing seems to be coming back also.

He told me not to worry, it was the change of weather and the flu season. I asked him to give the baby a flu shot. He told me that the baby was too young yet and even so, he could not give the baby flu shot because the baby was sick. He gave me a prescription for XOPENEX for another 14 days for his breathing (to be used with a nebulizer), and another prescription of CARBAXEFED DM for his coughing for 10 more days, and another prescription of **Amoxicillin 200 MG** for 14 days.

He said to me that this treatment was normal and done every day to all children. As I drove home, I was a bit worried about all the medicine, but knew that I was in no position to label this doctor's recommendation. I was not a doctor and he could easily report to DCF that I refused to medicate my grandson being in my custody; this is how cruel the medical community is today. At home, I started to see a change in our grandbaby; he did not play Peek-a-Boo anymore. His skin tone was not right, he started to look a little pale but he was eating OK at the time, and drinking his milk just fine. He started to dislike Amoxicillin, the antibiotic. He started to hate the taste of it but I had to give it to him as ordered by his doctor. I was not too worried because the doctor told me not to worry. I admit I was a little rusty playing daddy; after all, our children were adults. Here we were, our grandbaby was 8-months-old now and we cut a cake for him on his birthday. He did not smile much, was not playful anymore and pushed his cake over the high chair into the ground. I guess is because he had been sick for so long since December with his ears. Poor little baby I love so much; I never knew a baby could last so long with an illness but the doctor told me that it can last for months, so I must trust his care.

February 14th - on this visit, my baby still had his ears infected, and I was troubled because the baby had been on Amoxicillin all this time, a strong antibiotic, something just did not feel right. I tell Dr. Marlin that maybe he was right about the ear tubes. I suggested putting them in because the baby was not getting any better. He told me that it was still too early, and not to worry about the antibiotic, it will kill the ear infection as time goes by.

He told me that with some children it takes longer for the healing process, that he was the doctor and knows what is best. Having to hear that I just continued to follow his recommendations because he spoke with so much authority. I didn't want to find myself in front of the Department of Children and Family. At the time I was under the impression that these doctors can easily call the department of children and families, give a bad report card on you if you do not listen to them on behalf of your baby. This is a systematic DCF fear they put on parents if the child is somewhat involved with DCF. In this case, we only had custody of our grandbaby four months when we stepped into the Pediatric Clinic, and the doctor knew this. We had to believe and put all our faith in doctors before realizing any mishaps, which came after the fact in this case. I believe in back of every doctor's mind, inside a little closet in their head they believe they have the DCF Children & Family Power

Control Card over parents, so we had to be careful how we treat our doctors, but also try to be vigilant and wise.

We had no choice but to continue with Dr. Marlin's regimen of Amoxicillin. I was so ignorant at the time I just could not see what was really happening. He gave me another prescription of **Amoxicillin 200 MG**, but instead of 14 days, he gave it to me for 10 days and told me to come back to the clinic after the medication was used up, and was very demanding about it. He also gave me XOPENEX 0.63 MG for another 15 days for his breathing med. He did not give me anything for his coughing because the baby was doing a little better with his coughing.

<u>**February 24th**</u> - I went back to the clinic and I told Dr. Marlin that the ear infection had not gone away because the baby kept on grabbing the ears and on occasions, he cried. After the doctor examined the baby, he told me that the ears were starting to look better—that for now we would wait to see what happens. I was happy about that. I explained to him that his cough had come back; I told him that I still had some cough medication left, and then he checked my baby's chest and saw that my baby still had a breathing problem. I told him that I still had some XOPENEX left, and he told me to continue all medications.

<u>**March 8th**</u> - The baby did get plenty of bed rest, but still had the ear infection, and the coughing was getting worse and the fever would come and go. I decided to get a second opinion, so I went to another clinic. I did not know if I was crossing the line by taking my grandbaby to another doctor, but I started to get so worried that I needed a second opinion—after all he was my grandbaby. Therefore, I made an appointment to see Doctor Sandy in another clinic here in my town. I heard she was one of the best in town with children.

<u>**March 10th**</u> - I entered the clinic and met Dr. Sandy. She was pleasant and showed concern for my baby. She examined my baby and saw that he still had the ear infection in place to the fullest. After I told her about the clinic that I had taken my baby to, and the fact that the baby had been on Amoxicillin

since December, she showed concern but advised me to continue to go the original clinic I was going to. In this town, that clinic in question had a great reputation on curing children. She told me that in the past there last been other children like my baby that had taken a longer time to cure an ear infection, and not to worry because my baby was safe, that I should take the baby right now to his doctor. Well, upon hearing that I went straight back to the clinic that same day and saw Dr. Marlin again. His intern gave me another prescription for Amoxicillin 200 MG for 10 days, told me not to worry, that everything was going to be fine. He said he knew what he is doing, and after I finished the antibiotic not to get nervous but to let the medicine take its course. He also told me to buy some Tylenol for the fever instead of giving me another prescription for IBUPROFEN. That day was quite a day for me; after trying to get a second opinion with another doctor I just landed up right back where I started from, and with apparent high marks on Dr. Marlin and his clinic.

I felt a little embarrassed. I felt if though I was overreacting. After all I didn't know much about anything at the time, but I always got feedback from different people including my friends, saying that these pediatricians know what they're doing, so I had to stick it out. Therefore, I had to build some type of confidence and decided to have my baby tested for Early Prevention because he just did not want to play peek-a-boo. I did not want anything to interfere involving his growth because of all the Amoxicillin in his little body since Dec. 2004. I consulted with my wife on the matter and she agreed on the testing; she is more professional on the subject because of her teaching experience with child development pre-schools. She, of course, does not fail being on top of things.

March 23rd - The baby is 9 months old now, and today he will be tested. We had members from Early Steps Program, Division of Child Development and Neurology Department of Pediatric College of Medicine perform the testing. In the interview, I explained to the examiner of all the Amoxicillin— that it has me worried, and the fact that he does not play or does not have a happy face. That is the purpose for the testing. The examiner, who was a woman, explained to me that it is very good to do this testing on the baby at this age of 9 months, something she does not see often with other parents, even though she has tried to spread the message.

After the testing I was relieved to know that little Christopher passed all the exams for his age appropriate for 9 months old. It brought smiles to my wife and me. Poor little guy is going through some tough times and continues to remain sick. She explained to me that the child does not play or respond to certain things because the child is sick for the moment, and indeed, he is. Our minds were relieved, the joy in our hearts for that one moment felt so great.

March 28, still with the ear infection on Amoxicillin, all of a sudden the baby has developed a green pasty diarrhea, something out of this world. We got so nervous, so we go back to the clinic; this time they gave us Dr. Brunson, another pediatrician at the same clinic. I explained to Dr. Brunson all the problems, the diarrhea, that the baby is crying, still much in pain with his ears. I said his fevers come and go between 99 to 102. His coughing does not go away, but his breathing seems to be better. He explained to me that the problem here is that the antibiotic has been too weak, instead of giving the baby 200 MG, I am going to give him **Amoxicillin 600 MG** for every four hours for 10 days, and this should clear up his ears finally. However, as far as the diarrhea, he could not do anything about that because he has no prescriptions for diarrhea. I was to buy something over the counter to stop the diarrhea. For his fever, am to give the baby Tylenol and to continue the medication if he needs it for his breathing for which I had refills. I am starting to think that maybe I am living a dream, and the only way to wake up is to be punched in the face after talking with this doctor; I almost went out to look for someone, to do the job. Maybe I am behind the times if this is the way it is with doctors having power over Amoxicillin and children. My baby's green diarrhea lasted five days; imagine the discomfort plus all the crying and pain my baby went through.

April 4th - The baby started to get blood spots in his eyes. My heart fell to the ground when I saw the blood. I rushed back to the clinic without an appointment, and I saw Dr. Brunson again. He examined the baby's eyes, and said to me that the blood in the eyes is a natural thing that eventually will go away. I looked at him and asked him why my baby is going through so much all these months.

I am starting to get nervous. The doctor told me it was a good thing because he does not see that too often. Some babies take forever for the infection to end, and on my baby the infection was finally coming out. That is why I see his stool green and the blood reaction of the eyes. For a moment, I started to think about what he just said. It did not make any logical sense on this planet, but I just let it go because he was the doctor and I was stupid. He told me to continue the Amoxicillin. Again, I leave the clinic confused. That week my baby suffers more than ever because of his green diarrhea, the blood in his eyes, and I am going nuts. My wife and family are confused. Every day we all have family arguments over our grandbaby's sufferings. I felt our lives going upside down. It did not make any sense going to another doctor in this town because another had told me that it was O.K.

Things were not getting any better for my baby, but I had to trust these doctors and tried to tell my mind that everything was going to be fine. I had in my mind the testing I did back in March 23 on my baby that came out normal, so I just took a day at a time with the baby, which is all that was left for us. I felt our lives were full of confusion.

April 11th - I go back to the clinic, and this time they gave me Dr. Zoë, she is the head director of the clinic and she owns three other clinics here in town. I was happy about that; maybe this time she will take a different course of action for my baby. I explain to her all my concerns, everything the baby was going through, that maybe it's time for the ear tubes because the antibiotics are not working all these months.

I told her that the baby is teething and I was using Oral Jell for his teeth. She examined the baby and saw that the baby still had his ears infected. She told me to stop the Amoxicillin and she was going to prescribe another antibiotic OMNICEF 125 MG/5 SUS to be given to the baby for 10 days, then she tells me that the baby is doing fine— not to worry. I told her that we should put in the ear tubes. She told me it's impossible to put the ear tubes in because of the infected ears. She told me to follow her instructions—that everything was going to be all right. After I left the clinic, I started to get scared.

Two weeks passed now, and it is not pleasant for us. My baby now cries almost every day and it seems every time I picked him up for comfort it seems to work for a while but not for long, and it was getting worse by the minute. Our lives are infected with misery, our bills mount, the pressure is on, and we were never the same.

3
THE AMOXICILLIAN EXPERIMENT

April 25th - I went back to the clinic and was seen by Dr. Marlin himself, the baby's main doctor in this clinic. I told him that the baby still has the ear infection and cries a lot, grabbing on to his ears. I told him that the blood spots in the eyes are getting larger and that his breathing and coughing seems to be the same. His fevers come and go. He was puzzled and a bit upset.

He told me that he is going to try an experiment with the Amoxicillin. He said he is going to put the baby on Amoxicillin 400 MG every fourteen days straight without missing one dose for three months straight. I ask him if that is something normal because he has been on Amoxicillin almost five months now!

The doctor told me that my baby has a serious ear infection that few children develop, and that he is sure that after this experiment, that without any doubt the infection will subside. I asked him, "Won't that hurt the baby more than what the baby is going through?" He told me the medicine dose will not hurt the baby; it's the infection that hurts the baby. He is the doctor and I am just the parent. He said he knows what is best for the baby, to follow his recommendation to the letter. With that being said and with my baby being sick for the past five months, and him being a licensed MD pediatrician I totally believed in him, and he confirmed that he did this before. What choice did I have in the matter? I wanted my baby to be healthy again. He told me that he could not do anything about the blood spots in the eyes—that it was a normal thing, as they told me before.

He says that once the infection is out of the ears that he would then give me a referral to have the ear tubes be put in. Therefore, he gave me the prescription for Amoxicillin for three months, on top of the many months my baby had been on the drug already, and he told me not to miss a dose. He said to give the baby Tylenol for the fever and not to worry—that everything was going to be fine. The month of May, he was going to be away but I should have enough medicine for his condition for months to come.

June 8th, his birthday. Today he hits one year old. It is not much of a birthday for the little person; he spent his birthday in the crib crying all day, and we crying with him. We still bought him a cake and we blew out the candles for him. Our lives felt as though we were locked away from society, trapped in a cave, and the proprietor is the Devil himself.

Saturday June 11th, The baby gets the green diarrhea again, only this time it was more liquid than pasty and for a moment, we got scared, but then I remembered that he got the same diarrhea back on March 28th, so we thought nothing of it. We just put cream on his little butt. We still had some IMODIUM A-D left over for his diarrhea, so we gave him some. We were not worried because the doctor told us that mixing the medication would not hurt the baby. The next day in the afternoon the diarrhea was turning dark black green, something that did not occur back in March but we still did not think anything of it.

Monday June 13th, in the morning, it is a different matter, the diarrhea turns to an acid dark black green **with blood**, it was in liquid form. Blood! The baby was crying harder than ever. We went crazy. We dressed our baby and I run back to the clinic and saw Dr. Marlin again. He examines the baby and sees the bloody diarrhea that had a bad stench but tells me that there is nothing he could do about the diarrhea. "Continue to use the Imodium A-D and put cream for the rash."

He calmed me down by telling me that the diarrhea is green because the Amoxicillin is working, the infection is coming out of the baby finally. At the same time the baby is teething and that is what is causing the diarrhea. After hearing that I felt a little bit relieved. Then he tells me not to stop the regimen, to continue the Amoxicillin without stopping until the three months are up and to continue all the meds for his coughing if needed, but give the amoxicillin. I told him that the baby does not eat anymore, that he lost his appetite. He tells me to give the baby Pedialyte liquids so the baby does not dehydrate. I keep saying to myself that these doctors would not hurt babies or they would not be doctors. These were all the rationales that I keep putting in my mind, because these doctors are starting to scare me and my baby is not getting any better.

June 17th – It's been one week now and the baby still has the green bloody diarrhea, you could only imagine what my baby and my family went through that week. Not even the Imodium A-D is working, just changing diapers all day and every hour on the hour. Wish there was something I could do about the diarrhea so I decide to go back to the clinic to try to convince this doctor that there must be another way for the diarrhea to stop. Again, Dr. Marlin tells me that there is nothing he can do about the diarrhea, and he checks my baby again and finds that the baby still has the ear infection and to continue all the meds. That evening the diarrhea ended after seven days of misery, poor little guy.

July's Note: It's been almost eight months now that my baby has been on Amoxicillin, Carbaxefed cough medicine, Ibuprofen for fever, Tylenol for fever, Imodium A-D for diarrhea, and it has been not quite a year for my grandbaby living in pain and suffering, and being stuck with four crazy pediatricians in this small town. What to do with no end in sight? My wife does not seem well lately. She has come down with a few health concerns, and I have been over-exhausted with worry and tears almost every day myself. The baby does not eat anymore.

I am hardly eating myself, wondering when the baby is going to get well. In the month of July, I went to the clinic about five times, just back and forth.

The baby was just getting worse and worse, and these doctors just did not have any other options for my baby but only warnings for us, that we must follow their recommendations. It felt as though we were in some kind of nightmare with no return in waking up. Clinic from Hell!

July 19th We have another scary event seeing the baby's cough just get worse with a heavy hoarse sound. He starts to vomit, and his fever hits 103, so I go back to the clinic. Dr. Marlin examines the baby and sees that the baby has developed bronchitis. He tells me that he can not do anything for the vomiting, to continue the regiments of the Amoxicillin and that he is going to give my baby another antibiotic Omnicef 125/5 SUS for 10 days, the same antibiotic that the head director of the clinic gave me back in April. On that visit, the doctor gave me the impression that he was hiding something the way he looked at the baby after he examined him. I felt that something was wrong.

July 28th, 2005 would be the day that this pediatrician, Dr. Marlin, would finally give in to my concerns, finally! The baby's ears are still infected besides all the other problems with his breathing and coughing. He finally gives me a referral to put the ear tubes in after nine months of my baby's ears being infected, and me asking about the ear tubes. He finally does this because he realizes that his Amoxicillin Experiment is doing nothing but harming my baby throughout the year. After nine months of Amoxicillin 200 400 & 600 MG's, Xopenex 0.63 MG, Omnicef 125 MG antibiotic, fever medications, coughing medications—after all that Amoxicillin in my baby's system this doctor finally gives up his experiment. He tells me somehow he has to try to kill or slow down the infection first, before the ear tubes can be put in. He told me to stop giving the baby the **Amoxicillin 200 MG**, and he gave me a new prescription with refills for **Amoxicillin 600 MG**, a stronger dose to see if that would do the trick.

I explain to him that back in March Dr. Brunson gave me the same dose and it did not work, that is when Dr. Marlin said to me with all the amoxicillin in his body the 600 MG might work this time, to administer it for 10 days. He did not even know if this time the 600 MG, of Amoxicillin would work—just taking guesses. All we could do at that point was to go home and follow and continue his recommendations because the baby cannot get the ear tubes put in until the infection goes away. This small town is no good for rearing children. We just prayed to God every day that he would wake us up from this nightmare.

August Note: In the month of August, I would wind up visiting the clinic on emergency visits six times. The baby's skin color is starting to change and the fevers are starting to climb.

August 12th - Dr. Marlene saw my baby. This time I notice in the month of August on every visit Dr. Marlin, my grandbaby's main doctor is available, but ignores my baby and me on every visit in August. I feel that something is very wrong with his demeanor towards us. On this visit Dr. Marlene checks my baby and decides to give me a prescription for another antibiotic CEFZIL 125/5ML SUS for 10 days, and another type of cough medicine BROMAXEFED DM for 8 days.

August 25th, I see Dr. Zoë herself, head director and owner of the clinic. Just like all the other visits in the past, I explain to her all the problems as I did once before when I saw her months earlier, that my baby does not eat anymore etc, etc. I pleaded with her to try another option. Nevertheless, she defends her doctors that they know what they are doing, and she tells me that they are the doctors who know best for the child.

I tells her that the blood spots in the eyes are getting bigger. She says that there is nothing she can do about the blood spots, but not to worry because the blood spots will go away.

She tells me to continue feeding him Pedialyte for dehydration. She gave me another prescription for Amoxicillin 200 MG, for 15 days. I notice a rejection you might say coming from her towards my baby. She examines my baby too quick, too fast that day. The smell in the air was not right and it started to smell like my ignorance, how blind I was—and I felt hopeless. You would think Dr. Zoë, being head director, would take a different course of action, seeing that my baby's been on all these different medicines, especially the lengthy regimen of Amoxicillin for six months, and the Amoxicillin experiment for three months, making it nine months of Amoxicillin. Dr. Zoë would not take a different course of action. However, Dr. Zoë still decides to try to kill the ear infection through Amoxicillin, and scaring me with her authority.

It's hopeless; what do I do? I have to continue to listen to her because she is the doctor, and they keep throwing at me - that I do not want to hurt my baby, that I am just a caregiver, putting fear and negative thoughts in my mind. We are feeling that if we do not follow the doctors' orders that they will take our baby away because this is Florida where the laws are crazier than any other state in America. Florida, where over five hundred foster babies are unaccounted for (by now that number is higher).

The fighting and disagreements went on, day in day out with these doctors. The baby was getting worse. The expenses and our bills were growing by the minute and it seemed our world, as we knew it, was turning for the worse. It was nine months of pure hell seeing our baby deteriorating month after month in this Sebring Clinic of Horrors.

4
THE FINAL LAST DAYS

September Note: September would be the last month I would ever take my baby back to the clinic of horrors. September would be the last time these pediatricians would ever touch my baby. It's when I finally realized how wrong I had been in following these doctors' recommendations and listening to these doctors experimenting with Amoxicillin on my baby. How stupid I was!

Sept. 5th, Monday morning when I went to check on the baby, he was crying and in horrible pain. I walked over to his crib to pick him up for comfort, his crib mattress had a portion of blood underneath his bottom, coming out of the pamper. It was bloody acid. It was like a horror movie. His room smelled like a war zone of dead bodies.

My heart went to the ground; my wife was crying in agony. When we checked his pamper, he had the bloody black green acid diarrhea. We quickly cleaned him up and gave him some Imodium A-D to help try to stop the diarrhea. I started to think - back in June he had the same type of diarrhea, and it was a waste of time to go back to the doctor's office because back then they told me that there was nothing that they could do for the diarrhea. I acted calm and just concentrated on comforting the baby that entire day. I still had some Amoxicillin left for his ears; I saw no need to go to the clinic.

The next day, Sept. 6, was like a typical day of crying and pain; we had the medicine, we changed the diaper as much as possible to try to prevent diaper rash with the diarrhea. I did not know any better but to follow all the doctors' recommendations. I was stupid and a jerk and I ask God to forgive me every day of the week. I just had to prepare myself for all the extra pain and misery I was to endure. The next day hell was living in our grandson's room when we went into the room.

Wednesday Sept. 7th - Early in the morning the diarrhea turned to a liquid acid that burned right through the pamper with blood. It was incredible and there was a horrible smell like death in the diarrhea, so I quickly went straight to the clinic and was seen by Dr. Marlene. She examined and saw the bloody diarrhea, and his fever was 103, his ear infection has not gone away. I told her that he is not eating anymore, that I have him on Pedialyte liquids.

I told her that he needs to go to a hospital, that he does not look right. She quickly told me that will not be necessary; he does not need to be in a hospital. This will pass in the next day or two. She said that she is the doctor and she knows best. I asked her, "How about the bloody acid diarrhea?" She told me that she could not do anything about the diarrhea—that I should put cream on his butt for the rash. She told me to calm down. The diarrhea means the infection is coming out of him. She gave me another prescription for his coughing: Bromhist - PDX SYP for 7 days and she said to continue the Amoxicillin.

September 8th, I went back to the clinic because the baby did not sleep that night, crying the whole time in pain, and he was beginning to look worse, his fever hit 103 - 104, these were critical signs. This time it was Dr. Marlin and I saw in his face that he was nervous. He knew my baby was in trouble. The baby's bloody cheeks were hurting him a great deal. Dr. Marlin said that he was going to test the baby's stool at the lab in the hospital for any type of bacteria. I quickly got upset and asked, "What do you mean?" He explained to me that this is one of the testing's that he does on babies but only when it's called for.

So I yelled at him, "Then why wasn't this testing done back on June 4th three months ago when he first developed the same type of diarrhea? Or back in March, seven months ago when he first developed the green diarrhea?" The doctor had nothing to say regarding my questions, and then he gave me a bag to collect the stool so I could bring it to the hospital. He told me to continue the medications and asked me if I still had Amoxicillin?

I told him yes, because I still had some left from the prescription that Dr. Zoë gave me. I left that clinic very upset and saw how scared the doctor was. That afternoon I managed to collect the stool sample and quickly brought it over to the hospital, only to find out that the testing would not be complete for five days. I yelled at the personnel at Florida Hospital and told them that my baby might be dead by then, five days was too long! I thought to myself that Sebring, Florida, is the worst town in this country with crazy uncaring doctors, the worst in this country.

Friday September 9th, My baby's room smelled like death, same conditions in his crib with blood. He managed to get a little sleep the night before but I started to assume that the sleep only reflected his present weakness. However, I just had to go back to the clinic to let them know that the testing was not going to be ready for five days. They gave us Dr. Marlene and I told her that the bloody diarrhea did not seem to be changing, and the baby's fever seemed to hold at 104. I told her that yesterday Dr. Marlin had me go over to the hospital with a stool sample for lab testing but that it would take five days for the results. She looked at my baby's bloody cheeks and noticed the smell was horrible.

I told her that I was starting to worry about my baby's insides. Then she told me that she is worried about the alignment of my baby's stomach. She told me that she is going to recommend blood work and another stool sample that she is going to look for any other type of bacteria. I asked her the same question I asked the Dr. Marlin the day before; "Why wasn't this testing done months ago when he had the same symptoms of diarrhea?" She was very nervous and did not answer the question just as Dr. Marlin did not answer. These doctors knew that my baby was in trouble.

Again, I asked her whether maybe my baby should be admitted in the hospital. Again she told me "No" that he does not need to be in the hospital. She gave me a prescription for the blood testing and a bag for the stool, and told me to make sure I brought it to the lab that same day. She told me to continue all medications without stopping. For the fever, she told me to give him Tylenol every four hours and the next four hours after that to give him Motrin, and to repeat the process around the clock.

For the bloody cheeks, she gave me a prescription for a special cream Nystatin 100000U CRE for 10 days. She told me to put a layer of that cream, plus a layer on top of that cream of petroleum jelly as to make a thick wall base for the rash, and to block the blood from coming out of the pamper. I never saw these doctors more nervous and worried ever before; they all knew my baby was in danger.

That day I went to the local Florida Hospital with the stool sample, and at the same time, they gave my baby a blood test. It took four times of sticking the baby with the needle because they could not find a vein. My baby was suffering and crying in the process, and we were crying at the same time. My wife and I were going crazy to think that there are families with children moving into this crazy town, that even the hospital was causing our baby harm by looking for a vein by sticking the baby with the needle four times, playing guessing games. That day my baby was in more pain and suffering than ever before.

September 10th, the baby was not responding to anything, not even to a cry or a tear. His skin was pale and he did not recognize anything. The bloody diarrhea smelled even worse than death. Throughout the day we tried everything to grab his attention. Then in the late afternoon he awakened with a loud scream, crying in pain. Then he threw out the worst vomiting you can imagine. It was filled with blood. He vomited his guts out all over the entire floor in the living room.

We were so afraid that he was going to die, so we made the decision to take him to the emergency room at the hospital. We called all three local hospitals in this small town of Sebring, Florida, and none of them had the facility or capability of handling my baby's condition. They did not have a pediatric trauma emergency service for our children in this town. They told me that when we bring in the baby, at that time they would call a pediatrician.

They said that a pediatrician is just a phone call away. If at that time, a pediatrician feels he needs to be admitted they will fly him by helicopter to Tampa General. I yelled at them on the phone that my baby may die during all this loss of time for answers. That being said with all three crazy hospitals of this small town, we made the decision to call All Children's Hospital in St. Petersburg Florida. After speaking to the emergency room doctors from All Children's Hospital about my grandbaby's condition, and all of the things we went through they gave me an official order on the telephone to bring my baby into their emergency room ASAP or they were going to call the police. I told them on the phone that we were on our way the minute we hung up the phone. They asked me for my grandbaby's name and my name, and I gave it to them. The hospital was about 150 miles away. After I hung up the phone, we got the baby ready and prepared to leave.

Out of some crazy respect, I decided to call the answering service at my baby's pediatrician doctors, to let them know that we were taking the baby to the emergency room hospital at All Children's Hospital of St. Petersburg. Not one minute after I hung up the phone, as we are leaving our home the telephone rings... My wife made her way with the baby to the car. I picked up the phone and the caller was Dr. Marlene asking me what was going on?

After I told her our decision to take the baby to the hospital at All Children's of St. Petersburg, she got very upset and belligerent on the phone, yelling, "You have no right to do that! I am the doctor of the baby, if you want to go to the hospital; you should take him to Florida Hospital here in town. I will meet you there," she continued, "and if at that moment I feel that the baby should be admitted to the hospital, I will have the baby flown by helicopter to All Children's Hospital at St. Petersburg." I told her on the phone that I had strict orders from the hospital to take my baby into their emergency room

ASAP. Dr. Marlene then told me again as she has been telling me for months, that I'm just the parent but she is the baby's doctor, that I have to follow her advice. That is when I finally told her how wrong she and the other doctors were with my baby. As she kept talking on the phone interrupting me - I yelled at her and said, "Go *____* yourself, woman." I hung up the phone in her face, and then we left for the hospital with a bloody Grand-Baby hanging on to life. This is what happened to my baby in the hands of four lunatic Amoxicillin pediatricians in the Sebring Clinic of Horrors. That is what happened to my grandbaby, and I am ever so sorry my little Boo-Boo. May God Forgive Me……?

When I woke up from this deep zoned out episode of what had happened, my thoughts and vision were interrupted. The emergency room doctors came from the operation room to talk to me and my wife. We were nervous that the doctor would say he died. The doctor looked at us and said, "Christopher will live, the danger is over!" However, we still had to wait awhile longer before we could see our baby. He said, "Just hang in there.

I looked at the doctor and said "God bless you. Thank you." I hugged my wife in tears, my wife crying in my arms. It was great news. We hugged each other and just sat motionless, we just sat there in tears with a joyful heart. I started to remember about the Amoxicillin experiment plus the Amoxicillin long-term regimen they gave my baby for those nine months. How stupid and blind was I to put my 100% trust and confidence in these doctors when it came to my baby's health.

5
THE DISCHARGE

I sat there in All Children's Hospital Emergency Room waiting to see my grandson. After nine months of misery, pain, and torture now today my baby's lifeless body was being saved by All Children's Hospital. One could only surmise that everything is going to be fine for Christopher; but that is not the case.

I grabbed my wife very hard in tears, praying to God that the doctors who were working on him now can tell us if he will be all right in the near future. He is in bad shape and lost a lot of blood driving over here, and he had the smell of death on him. They had been working with him for two hours now. A nurse came over to comfort us and gave us a small bottle of water.

She looks at me and says not to worry because the best thing we did was bringing the baby to this hospital. All they do here is work with children, and the doctors here are top specialists. She was kind and professional and I started to think positively but could not help wondering what the baby must be going through right now. Suddenly, a doctor came from the room and told us that it's O.K. to go see our baby. The joy glowed from our faces with tears like Niagara Falls. So we hopped to it. As we approached our baby, we were just crying and saw that he was not crying but just in a sleeping state. He had IV tubes going on his arm and his mouth. They told us that the blood in the diapers came from the black liquid acid diarrhea that peeled off the skin from his butt cheeks, and the blood was coming from the skin mixing with the diarrhea.

That is why the blood was coming down his legs, and the blood at the house in his bed was from the same condition. The acid diarrhea was so strong that it also was burning through the diapers and most probably through his bed sheets; they told us that this might be his last episode of acid bloody diarrhea. The IV and meds he was getting would do away with that. They also had another tube going into the baby's other arm for special antibiotics and the other was an IV for food.

The doctor told us that the baby was dehydrated beyond the norm and was at a danger level. They were waiting for lab results, but they believed the baby had a few types of bacteria that were destroying the baby's system. The doctor told us after the lab work was completed; they could determine what type of bacteria was shutting down the baby's system. They said one thing was for certain: giving a baby Amoxicillin for the lengthy time period of nine months was crazy in their viewpoint, and a death sentence for the baby was imminent with this type of treatment. The danger came from the nine months of Amoxicillin inside the system of a baby; it was crazy and deadly. They also had a heart monitor set up in front of the baby's bed. It was about 2:30 am Sunday morning and the hospital made us as comfortable as possible. About 3:00 am, they came in to transfer the baby from the emergency room to a private room upstairs in one of the pediatric wards.

It was just heartbreaking seeing the attendant wheeling our baby to a private room. The hospital was big, with cartoon pictures all over the walls and elevator, a reassurance that my baby came to the right place. We could not sleep at all that night, though they had sleeping recliners for us in the room. A night nurse monitored our baby through the night. At about 8:00 am that morning a team of seven doctors came to the bedside of my baby. One was the Dr. Christina, in charge of my baby, and she introduced the other doctors that were in training.

Dr. Christina asked me about my baby, and I told her about the nine months of my baby being on so much Amoxicillin and other antibiotics, besides breathing medicines. I told her of the dark green, black looking bloody acid diarrhea. I could see the other doctors looking at my baby's chart as I was talking. My baby's doctor read the chart and told me that once the lab testing was complete that she would return to speak with us, that for now the baby was stable and doing fine—-that we should not worry. Then she looked at the team of doctors and started to talk to them about my baby's chart. I could not hear or rather I did not pay attention to them, but I could see the concern that some doctors had on their faces over my grandson's chart. At about 10:00 am, the baby woke up, looking at us with a cry, wondering where he was and what was going on as he looked at the needles in his arm. We quickly started to wipe his tears and give him as much love and concern as possible so he would not be afraid. Then we started to cry with him. I took out the portable DVD player and played his favorite DVD - Dora. The nurse came in to change the IV and he got frightened and started to cry in fear just looking at me.

It was if he was saying - "Help me, poppa," and I felt so hopeless in coming to his rescue not only in that moment, but also in the past ten months. I was mentally destroyed at that moment. At about 1:00 pm that afternoon Dr. Christina walked in with the results of the lab testing. She said that the baby suffered from strains of bacteria growing in his digestive tract, and his immune system, slowly shutting down his body, could have killed him if we did not bring him to the hospital.

My heart went to the ground after hearing that. She said to us that the baby lost too much body fluid and blood, and had too much diarrhea that dehydrated him, all because of the amount of Amoxicillin in his system for a baby. She says too many antibiotics in the baby's system for such a long period of nine months was dangerous, lethal, and deadly for any baby.

The diagnosis for Chris - (1) Dehydration, (2) Clostridium Defficile bacterium, (3) Acute Gastroenteritis, (4) Chronic Otitis, plus the bloody butt cheeks, (5) C-Difficille toxin B. My baby was suffering from all this bacteria in his system all these months. The doctor told us he would be staying at all children's hospital until he is well enough to go home. We brought the baby on time to the emergency room; she also said one more day and it would have been over for the baby, and we did well in bringing him to the hospital. Then she told us in a low tone "Your baby is out of danger but will have complications in the future. We cannot say what type of complications but it will be developmental."

This, of course, was bad news for us. We asked her what she meant that he "might later have developmental issues to deal with." She could not get any deeper than that about what she meant, but just told us to watch him closely and to prepare ourselves for his future, regarding how much damage was done to the baby. My tears just kept coming down my face. My wife looked at me and said to me in tears - "Whatever it takes, we will help our baby until we die!" We hugged in tears and the baby went fast asleep. She also told us that Christopher is one remarkable baby with an unbelievable will to live.

The relief off our shoulders was that the baby was going to live. After all these months of pain it was nice to see him sleeping peacefully, but it hurt to know where he landed after that peaceful sleep. The nurse came back into the room and shared with us the accommodations where we could stay free of charge. It was a McDonald House type hotel that the hospital and McDonalds made available to the children's parents. The location was right next door to the hospital, which was great. I was very impressed with how they treated my baby and us in this hospital. My wife started to tell me about the wonderful things that the Ronald McDonald House has been doing for years. She knew about this service through her known parents. As my wife stood watch in the room, I decided to take a walk through the floors of the hospital. I noticed how everything is designed only for the children; it was a great feeling seeing all these children being cared for at the right hospital. I noticed as I walked by some of the children's rooms, the sadness was in the air.

I also saw the happiness the parents expressed seeing their babies are cared for—it was a warm feeling I felt. Each child was there for a different reason. Some rooms had two beds and some had only one. I noticed my grandbaby only had one bed also in his room. I asked a nurse why that was? She told me that the children who were alone in the room had a contagious illness. I did not know that. So I went back to the baby's room thinking to myself, "Will the baby pull through all this?"

I felt even worse inside now that I knew his illness was contagious, poor little baby. My mind was thinking negatively about everything; positivity flew out the window. He must have had a strong will to live because he survived, and I was proud of him for that. Days passed, and every day he showed signs of getting better. On the third day, we had a little party in his room. He was alive with joy, and his ear infection had gone away after almost ten months of suffering, but his stool was still green with no diarrhea, and his eyes still had a little blood with blood spots. His fever was gone, and we were happy. That afternoon the doctor gave us the heads up that the baby could leave tomorrow, and that was great news because we started feeling like a hospital within our bodies. My grandbaby was in the hospital for four days. Discharged on September 14. 2005, he looked so good and started to smile for the first time since we could remember. On the day of discharge they gave him some stuffed animals and wheel chaired him out of the hospital.

All the nurses were smiling with him; it was a beautiful day. The doctor told us that the dehydration was gone. They explained to us what we needed to do for the baby, - discontinue the Amoxicillin, no milk for a while, give yogurt twice or three times a day, and avoid apple juice or any juice with high sugar. The blood spots in the eyes were never going away, the blood spots were there to stay. They asked us to call them back if the baby started vomiting, had diarrhea, or any other type of problem.

We had to bear in mind that his stool would remain green for a very long time into the future. It might go away and it may come back green. His immune system has been compromised so much with antibiotics, it created an alteration to his system; this would be the reason for his stool being green. Even though they did a great job for my baby, I had this feeling inside of me that from now on I would never trust any doctors, no matter what. They gave us some information on the C-Defficile bacteria. However, I have to admit that everything that was said to me at the hospital and all explanations on my baby's condition sounded like German. I just did not understand the diagnosis on my baby but knew that it must have been bad, and I had to take time to learn and educate myself for the future of my grandson. However, besides being happy for his discharge, I was also very upset and could not wait to get home. As we started to head home from the hospital, the baby was sleeping in the car seat and my wife told me that we cannot let those doctors get away with this, and hurting any other child for that matter.

Of course, I agreed, but I knew that the road ahead was going to be complicated because the doctors in question were well known in this little town, so it would have to be an attorney from outside the town. So here we are driving home, after spending four days in the hospital saving my baby's life. I started thinking of what the doctors in the hospital told me - Christopher was going to have problems in the future.

I guess we were going to have him tested again, as we did when he was 10 months old while on antibiotics with the Early Steps Program. Imagine that for a moment - I had the baby tested when he was 10 months old because we were scared about all the antibiotics in his system back then. We were hoping that he passed all his motor skills tests. Now he landed in the hospital almost dead, came out of the hospital with doctors telling me that he was going to have developmental issues.

If this is true, I would have him tested again, for his motor skills in-depth testing. His future would be expensive and our lives would change forever! We finally reached our home. As we entered our driveway, the baby all of the sudden woke up with a smile. He was still dramatized with everything around him. After we settled in with the baby, wife and I started to write down everything that we needed to do. First, the baby would need a new pediatrician MD.

Second, we had to find out if the doctors from All Children's Hospital were right about the doctors in question having no right to give a 6-month-old baby nine months of Amoxicillin. Third, we had to find out all the medical information I could on all of the baby's diagnoses that almost killed him. I quickly went to visit the doctors that put my baby in the hospital. As I entered the clinic I noticed the parents and the children sitting in the waiting room, my thoughts of sorrow just poured out to all of them. I walked up to the window and said hello to the secretary and notice that Dr. Marlin was on the other side.

The secretary said hello. The doctor did not say anything; none of them asked about Christopher's health. I quickly said to her that I was there for my grandbaby's medical records. She, of course, was surprised, and told me that she would have to find time to do the job, and that I may have to pay $1 dollar a sheet. I could not believe it, they would charge for a piece of paper with my grandbaby's information? I told the secretary that I would wait and would pay cash for the copies. After I received the copies, I went to work researching all that night. It was going to be a long night. I then prepared the baby's pedialyte electrolyte drink. We gave him that instead of milk because we could not give him any milk for a while. The pediatric electrolyte drink restored the body's water, minerals, and electrolytes, keeping the baby from dehydration. We hoped the destruction within the baby's system would be reconstructed in due time, if it was even possible.

6
THE NIGHTMARE BEGINS AGAIN

Two days after Chris was discharged from the hospital, the baby's nightmare began again. In the early morning hours of Sept. 17, we could hear a yell from the baby's room. I ran to the room and my wife began to "scream" and so did I. The baby's bed was filled with black acid diarrhea and blood again, and the baby was frighten and scared. My wife yelled at me to call the hospital again.

I picked up the baby and moved him over to the living room where the phone was located. As I started to dial the number the baby gave a big scream and vomited a great deal. The vomit had a littler blood, and it was all over the floor. I gave a big scream to my wife for help. I dropped the phone and told the baby not to worry. My wife came with a couple of wet towels; I quickly grabbed the phone and called the hospital.

I told them what was happening; again, they gave me another order to bring in the baby to the emergency room at once. The drive to the hospital was no different from the first time. We just did not have an escort. So here, we go again in the same condition of having to make short stops to change the burning acid diarrhea diapers on a long ride on the highway. A two-hour drive converted to about four hours because it was the morning rush hour, and I had to stay focused as much as possible and believe that everything was going to be O.K. I was driving like a midday mad driver. However, I was extra cautious; maybe that is why the police never noticed me. I noticed in the rear view mirror the baby crying in pain, and my wife doing a great job in comforting the baby in her own tears. I was just pounding on my head with confusion, why was this happening to my grandbaby. Why was this happening to us?

Once we arrived at the hospital they took him and admitted him immediately again on September 17 for the second time. Unbelievably, we just left this hospital three days before and now we were back. Again, they hooked the baby up to an IV for dehydration. It was unbelievable how much vomit came out of his mouth—like a horror movie. The doctors could not believe that we were back. Even they looked a little upset. They took the pampers that had the diarrhea for lab testing, and took our baby upstairs to another room.

My baby was again in shock and crying all day, because he did not want to be in the hospital. He was only 15 ½ months old with 9 months of pain and suffering. This time we were more scared than ever; now we were back to the drawing board. Of course, he looked more alive than the last time we brought him in. Again, we checked into the Ronald McDonald's House next to the hospital. This time poor little Christopher was diagnosed with Rotavirus AGE, and still had the C-Defficile bacteria & bloody stool diarrhea with high fever. This time they kept him at All Children's Hospital for another five days. Of course, we also spent every day and night at the hospital and took turns going back and forth to the Ronald McDonalds House to take showers, as we did when he was here last week. We were just in another world and the nightmare did not leave our baby. It killed me inside to see him like this, days on end in this hospital with no end in sight. The first couple of days were misery for my baby in the hospital, just like the first time. On the third day, he started to slow down his crying, and the nurses did a wonderful job with the baby.

On the fourth day, he was playing with his hands with Mama in a crib that looks like an incubator, because the virus the baby is carrying was contagious just like last week, with the same bed but a different room. It was a beautiful sight seeing Mama smiling with Boo-Boo. As the days passed Boo-Boo started to show signs of recovery, and it was apparent to me that he was doing great.

The doctors came into the room and said that he was out of danger, and they showed their sorrow that we had to bring the baby back to the hospital. I did not blame the hospital for my baby's return because, after all, his system was destroyed. The rotavirus was under control but the stool would remain as they told us the last time. It would be green for years to come. The diarrhea was gone, and he was a happy child once again. On the day of September 23 it was time for his second discharge in two weeks. All Children's Hospital did a good job in explaining everything regarding the baby's needs. The doctor told us not to forget to make an appointment to have ear tubes put into the baby's ears.

The ear tubes were something that my baby's ex-pediatricians who put him in the hospital should have done months ago, before the massive destruction took place in my baby's system. The doctor said to me that the baby would need our attention around the clock, seven days a week for years to come.

She told us that she could not say when his developmental change would take affect, and in what form, but for what the baby had been through, it was a miracle that he survived. As I was driving home, I started to think everything the doctors at the hospital told us over the two week span. I learned allot and had so much to learn still. But I also learned how stupid of a man I truly was. Underneath this macho attitude of mine, I felt stupid not to have known the most important things that would touch my baby's life along his way toward growth.

I should have known that the baby would have gotten ear infections along the way. I should have known about the Amoxicillin and other antibiotics, and the damage it causes babies internally. I should have known the history of Amoxicillin. I should have known that pediatricians are not up to par when it comes to the latest news and research on Amoxicillin that may and will affect our children's future forever. I should have known that you do not experiment with Amoxicillin on a child. What these pediatricians did by making me shove down my baby's throat 34 cycles of Amoxicillin in 9 months was lethal and deadly. The hospital was in disbelief to learn of the 34 cycles. In addition, I should have known that the doctors that treated him surely knew the dangers of Amoxicillin, because they knew the side affects were deadly. I should have known not to put all my trust in doctors, who care more about money and insurance than for my baby, and I should have never followed the doctor's orders, but I did!

For that, I will always hate myself. A small 6-month-old baby on nine months of amoxicillin in his little body, over an ear infection that just did not want to go away with Amoxicillin. These doctors just did not want to lose the battle with their Amoxicillin experiment against my baby's ear infection, so they decided to cross the line, and that crossing endangered my grandbaby's life forever. What is done cannot be changed, but the outcome of what is done can be learned with love and compassion, to see a better tomorrow for his life.

After the hospital experience, the first order of business was to make an appointment for the baby's ear tubes. I had to find a new pediatrician MD for the baby, and make an appointment with the Early Steps Children Medical Services. When the baby was nine months old, we had him tested for his motor skills because we started to see that the baby just did not play or respond to patty cake or anything for that matter. Most of the time he was just crying when he was nine months old.

Even with all the Amoxicillin that he was taking at the time, and all the crying he was doing, Christopher passed his motor skill testing at nine months with excellence. Today, however, from this moment on into the future it would be a different matter. The doctors told us at the hospital how crazy it was for any pediatricians to prescribe such an amount of antibiotic into any baby's system. They told us that he was going to have developmental issues and for us to give him our full attention 24 hours a day 7 days a week, putting our lives in a different direction with God's help.

They also told us not to blame ourselves—that we were following the doctors' orders and we should not hold ourselves accountable. It was nice of them to try to make us feel better, but yes, I do blame myself but will not let that pain ruin my life. I must still make important decisions in my life. Finally, the day came when Christopher was going to have the ear tubes put in, one month after he left the hospital.

He was 16 ½ months old. It would be a very small surgical procedure. Of course, when I heard that, I wanted to know what kind of procedure? Were there any other options besides the ear tubes, and most of all is there pain involved? My baby had been through enough pain and misery for nine months straight. The Surgeon explained to us that it would be a very tiny tube as small as a grind of sand. The tube is placed inside the ear canal through a small slit in the ear that they perform through a surgical procedure. The procedure takes about 10 to 15 minutes. What the tube will do is to drain out any fluids, even pus that is harmful for the baby's ears. The fluid drains out of the ear with the help of the tube. This, of course, is a great help and has a good track record of helping millions of children with ear infections. However, I have to tell you it was not easy for Boo-Boo the day we took him to the hospital for the operation; it brought him bad memories.

He could not speak at the time on that day, but the expression on his face said it all and he broke down in a meltdown. The meltdown lasted a lengthy time, but he came through it. After the 15-minute operation the surgeon told us that Boo-Boo would not have ear infections anymore—no more pain, because the fluids would be drained. I felt a great heavy relief off my shoulders and mind, but still worried about the future for Boo-Boo. After the operation, Boo-Boo came out smiling as if he did not know that he was operated on.

As time passed, he had no more ear infections; he was finally free from ear infections after eleven straight months of an ear infection, nine of those months through the pain and torture of Amoxicillin and Bacteria shutting his body down… Since he left the hospital, our time with Boo-Boo has been much closer than we ever imagined.

We think of him all day and night and we do everything with him; and we notice, with his beautiful smile, how secure he truly feels now. That smile makes me feel good and keeps me going for his benefit. Now it was time to make an appointment for the baby to see if his development had been altered in any way. I sat there thinking of how I was going to repair the damage that was done to my baby. However, one thing was for sure right now, that my baby was put in the hospital in the condition that he was in due to his pediatricians Amoxicillin treatments and experiments. Every day is a challenge facing new information on Autism & Developmental Delay. The more I can get information, the more I can help our baby. For him it's a new frontier, and for us it's a different challenge, one that we have to welcome whether we like it or not because we love him. It is love that will see us through all the hardships that we are about to face and the facts that lie ahead.

7
RECIPE FOR AUTISM

It is without question that our children may need treatment or an antibiotic to kill off infections when the moment occurs. It is also without question they do have other methods to draw off infections less dangerous for our children. I am not going to tell you which antibiotic is best for your children; I am not a doctor.

I will say this: ask your pediatricians to put your children on medicine that will not damage or injure the children's system through random consumption of the same antibiotic # 1 Amoxicillin. Those years, 2006 into 2008, my grandbaby went through an in-depth training through Early Steps program, plus speech therapy because he could not speak a word. Also he had training in motor skills, occupational therapy, and potty training, because he just did not know anything, even after constant training.

He was going to a neurologist at All Children's Hospital for the twisting of his hands and other disorders. The right and left hands twist upward when he is upset because he gets mad when he doesn't understand or can't comprehend things around him, then he goes into long meltdowns. These are just some of the changes he has to adjust himself to, as well as us his family. I also have to adjust to his new world of survival because everything will be confusion; he will not recognize bullying. His grandmother and I worked endlessly around the clock 24 hours 7 days a week of the year with him. My wife who is an early head start teacher has done wonders beyond the call of duty. Sufferings have hit us like no other disasters we can think of. We suffer a great deal and have changed our way of life for baby Christopher. We buried ourselves in debt with constant supplies and things we had to buy for him to make his life more comfortable.

I cannot even imagine the millions of children with Autism and their parent's expenses for their children. It is very expensive to raise these children with disorders the right way, but we should not care about that. God will reward you for your work in taking good care of his children and your baby. On his birthday June, 2006, he was two years old, and he was jumping in joy. He had a beautiful smile, all the children were around him, and it was a wonderful sight. Just to think, months earlier he was in the hospital almost dead with bloody acid diarrhea, and all kinds of bacteria eating him up inside.

He may not speak or potty or be like the normal child but I have him alive and that is what counts. That day my wife and I spoke, it was time to seek legal action against these doctors. But I felt that we needed more time with Christopher because of his meltdowns around the clock. That year all my energy went to my grandson after witnessing what he went through in torture and pain with the Amoxicillin. He needed us every minute of the day with no interferences. Then everything changed on September, 2006, four months after his birthday. He was 28 months old, did not speak a word yet and he had an appointment with the Neurologist at All Children's Hospital. After all the testing was completed it was a sad day for us to learn that he was diagnosed with Developmental Delay and Autism. This of course would account for many different problems he has demonstrated, including his meltdowns the twisting of his hands, lack of social communication, and mind zoning out episodes.

This puts a dent on all the hard work that we have done with Christopher. Now it was time for a new setting, for a more complex challenge regarding his future. My mind went into limbo again just thinking of how normal he was the first six months on this planet, and the torture he had been through nine months after that—all because of an ear infection that did not want to go away, and the 9 months of Amoxicillin that almost killed him.

I had stood in a corner, feeling hopeless, without any power to give him the justice that he needed. This made me more furious, so I did an in-depth research on Autism Spectrum Disorder and Developmental Delay. My guard was up, and I went to work. Night after night, day after day, non-stop I tried to learn why a healthy boy, who is born normal, turns out to be autistic from Amoxicillin. After my final research, I have never been so disgusted with our medical community and our government. They have allowed the creation of the Amoxicillin Autism Affect to take hold of our children.

The high rising number of children infected with Autism today, for me plays a big role allowing pharmaceutical companies, lawmakers, money, power and control over our children's health care; and profit is the foundation of their motive for creating this drug. They heard the cries of parents back in the 80's about their new drug, amoxicillin, changing their children's development, but the pharmaceutical companies ignored them, as did our own government's Dept. of Health.

One thing that I noticed through all the testing since Christopher came out of the hospital being diagnosed with developmental delay and autism spectrum disorder. Though I saw many different doctors and his new pediatrician, not one of them voiced their opinion regarding the fact that Amoxicillin caused my baby's autism. Until this day, every doctor I know will shy away from the topic of amoxicillin, saying it is impossible.

Moreover, not once did any of these current doctors who have been treating my baby for autism, dare to tell me or even suggest that my baby may have gotten his autism from genetic or environmental reasons after hearing the story of amoxicillin causing my baby's autism. Why? I assume after what I know, I can say that some doctors know too well about the 20-cycle limit of amoxicillin in a child's system. They know it's the borderline to altering children's development. They know that the 34 cycles in nine months of Amoxicillin that almost killed my baby was crazy coming from four pediatricians. They knew that their peers in child healthcare should be terminated from practice. I believe every doctor knows that Amoxicillin is the perfect recipe for Autism. This negligence of doctors feeding Amoxicillin to a level of danger with no return is the leading cause for the millions of children in America being diagnosed with autism. While talking to these pediatricians who did this to my baby, reading their body language indicated that they know amoxicillin ruined my baby's immune system, and compromised his intestines.

This is an alteration that caused my baby's developmental delay problems in his mind, among many other disorders he is experiencing as he grows older. None of these caring professionals—pediatricians or medical doctors, has the decency to come out and say - "that indeed it was the Amoxicillin Experiment of nine months that caused the development of autism in my grandbaby. The emergency room doctors at All Children's Hospital that saved his life confirmed that indeed our baby was not going to be the same anymore.

I believe is like a contract that pediatricians have to protect the pharmaceutical companies and the medicines they prescribe to parents. However, now it's a different matter. Whether they like it or not, they are going to hear the truth, and the truth is the Amoxicillin Autism Affect is real and is here to stay. The Amoxicillin Autism Affect has been in existence for the past 30 years since the introduction of Amoxicillin. I am contending that the great majority of 1 in 88 children come from being born without any complications. Then in later years through the consumption of so many cycles of amoxicillin through the first five years of their lives the amoxicillin autism affect takes place. What hurts so much is that the research has been done on Amoxicillin and other antibiotics that cause this disease. The medical community knows the link with Amoxicillin and Autism, because they heard this story 30 years ago from parents whose children's today are adults with autism; surviving this cruel way of life.

This explosive recipe works on the child's brain development first, and as time continues to pass, the parents do not know anything. As you continue giving your children Amoxicillin for their sicknesses, then disorders start to form in the child because the damage is growing greater by the day within the child's system. Studies were done after seeing the numbers change from 1 in 10,000 to 1 in 166, to 1 in 150 to 1 in 100 to 1 in 88 today.

The reason you do not hear about these positive studies against amoxicillin is because they refuse to accept it. The drug is a Billion Dollar Profit Giant. The people have the authority regarding their children, and we must demand no more prescribing amoxicillin to our children. They must come back with a safer drug. Do not take my word for it, do your research, and get on the band wagon to stop these doctors and the big honchos—-the CEO's of these pharmaceutical companies who have control over Amoxicillin that is killing our children slowly. I ask all you good parents to write letters to the government's Health Dept. and to the President after you realize the truth of the matter.

Anyone that even thinks I'm barking up the wrong tree—that I just decided one day to attack the pharmaceutical companies and Amoxicillin—is very wrong about that. I just did not get up one day and say, "Hey, I want to be a famous writer today to sell books against the antibiotic, Amoxicillin." Forget about it! No,

I woke up one day and saw my grandson's anatomy changing and his mind altered due to your amoxicillin, and I said, "Hey, today I'm going to let the world know how irresponsible the medical community has been to our children for the past 30 years. My problem is the introduction of Amoxicillin to pediatricians, making it the #1 antibiotic for babies and children, which almost killed my grandbaby and have killed others. A drug caused harm to millions of babies and children in this country, and the numbers keep rising. Look at some of these things that have happened to my grandbaby, and hear for yourself what some researchers and their study have found.

Fact: - My baby was born a normal playful baby until he was six months old when he had an ear infection. He was put on Amoxicillin that lasted nine months straight for an ear infection that did not want to leave. During those nine months, his system was shutting down; he was suffering and could not speak to tell me what was wrong.

Nine months of this drug caused my baby bloody diarrhea, breathing problems, vomiting, and many red flags indicating bacteria and his doctors did not even care to do proper testing. No stool samples or blood work was done until the last week of his dying days. At the same time, the Amoxicillin was destroying his immune system, making the drug resistant to the ear infection, and killing all the good bacteria as well as the bad bacteria, landing him in the hospital almost dead at 15 ½ months old with his insides damaged and altered.

Fact: After the baby came out of the hospital, our baby was seen by a Pediatric Neurologist from the same hospital. They themselves diagnosed our baby with autism developmental delay. Question is, how did he contract this disease? For the logical minds who are reading this story, it is obvious that the Amoxicillin landed him in the hospital and destroyed the baby's system. Before the baby was discharged the doctors themselves in the hospital told me that his development was going to be a major problem and to prepare ourselves for the outcome. We parents must put an end to the use of Amoxicillin that is infecting our children, and this is the answer.

The proof is clear, the evidence of my son to the Amoxicillin Autism Affect. It was a thirty-year recipe with a track record of success altering our children's minds, and my concern and fear is that many future newborns may experience that same fate. It's time to put up a stop sign. Stop hurting our children with this antibiotic that is damaging their immune system and other vital organs that contribute to the development of Autism. This Stop sign will happen and will appear someday! 'You want more, here are some powerful studies I believe to be true with similar affects to what my baby went through during his nine months of amoxicillin, and is going through today. I say these studies hit home in the hearts of all parents.

Fact: A powerful survey was done over twenty years ago that would have saved some millions of children from contracting Autism, Developmental Delay today. It would have started the recovery process of cutting down the production we see in children being diagnosed with autism today. If the medical community would have done something about the complaints coming from parents and taken these studies seriously, our children would not be suffering with this disease. The study was done by the Developmental Delay Registry a Multi-National Database of 800 families at the time, most of whom had children with developmental delays and Autism.

The nine-month survey began in June, 1994, which included youngsters between the ages of one year old and twelve years of age. It found that those who had taken more than 20 cycles of antibiotics in their lifetime (1 to 12 years old) are over 50% more likely to suffer and contract Developmental Delays. My grandbaby had 34 cycles of Amoxicillin in nine months fed to his system turning him developmental delay, and Autism today.. With this study by the Developmental Delay Registry, I say that my grandbaby contracted Autism from the Amoxicillin of 34 cycles that his small tiny body had to endure. This was far more dangerous than the study of 20 cycles within a twelve-year period. However, the study also shows children who have only had fewer cycles of Amoxicillin or any other antibiotic were half as likely to become developmental delayed. This is evidence you cannot deny from this survey in connection with the subject matter. In my opinion as a parent, the medical community and our government, as well as pharmaceutical companies stating the excuse of needing more evidence on amoxicillin is bogus.

It is all about continuing the money river floating into their purse until the time limit is up. When that time comes, we will see in this country 1 in 10 children being diagnosed with autism. My friends, children in this country are on the receiving end of so many antibiotics, especially the number one drug, amoxicillin—the drug of choice by pediatricians all over this country. The biggest disturbing link are those children using Amoxicillin every day, and parents not realizing the possible injury and brain damage they're doing to their children as demonstrated by this survey.

Fact: - The study showed over 20 cycles to the danger level. My grandbaby was given 34-cycles in nine months and survived from some of these deadly bacteria's, C-Difficille Bacteria, Rotavirus Bacteria, to name a few. Baby had bloody diarrhea, bloody eyes, vomiting, weight loss, his immune system completely compromised along with his intestinal tract, destruction of his good bacteria as well as his bad. The nationwide survey that has been ignored dealt with over 700 children. It showed a disturbing link between children with developmental delays and the amount of Amoxicillin they had taken into their system, as administered by parents with prescriptions from pediatricians. The study showed that 75% of the Delayed Children were reported to be developing normally in their first year of life; just like in my baby's case. After that first year is when my baby started to reflect developmental complications on this antibiotic. Other findings in the survey showed 37% of developmentally delayed children were more likely to have had three or more ear infections than the unaffected children that did not have developmental delay problems.

Affected children from amoxicillin were twice as likely to have ear tubes as the unaffected children were. For the doctors and researchers that are protecting Amoxicillin, I say put an end to the production of Autism in this country by stopping this flow of Amoxicillin. My grandbaby is living proof of the survey that was introduced by the Developmental Delay Registry in 1994. Shame on the medical community and shame on our Government for ignoring such a powerful survey that would have saved millions of children today.

The survey hit it on the head because my baby was born normal. My baby was doing fine until his ear infection at the age of 6 months, but his pediatricians decided to alter his normal development through 9 months of Amoxicillin. Millions of children have developed autism at different ages between 1 and 12, and if you feel that your child may be part of this amoxicillin dilemma, then find out from your pediatrician how many cycles of amoxicillin your child has taken since birth. The parent can tell if their child is part of the Amoxicillin Autism Affect. This is one way to identify the source of your child's autism. Most of our children may have been victims of this amoxicillin recipe but we just don't know. You can also get a history of your child's cycles of amoxicillin from your pharmacist; even from Wal-Mart. Wal-Mart will give you a printout.

Remember a cycle is a treatment of amoxicillin 7 or 10 days per cycle. It is said that twenty cycles is at the norm between 1 to 12 years of age. It is sad to see more than 20 cycles on a child in less than 5 years. This is evidence you cannot deny on how children today and my baby developed autism. Here is a warning from a nutritionist:

Fact: - Kelly Dorfman, Licensed Nutritionist and Co-Founder of the Developmental Delay Registry. She cautions - "Parents should be put on notice that utilizing antibiotics like Amoxicillin prophylactically could jeopardize their children's development, alternative approaches to treating ear infections should be considered." I put all my trust in the pediatricians and the Amoxicillin they recommended for nine months, hurting my baby without even knowing it. But they knew about this danger. The medical community that is protecting Amoxicillin and other antibiotics will disagree with anyone who claims amoxicillin causes autism. I say this is evidence I cannot deny!

Fact: Since the introduction of Amoxicillin to pediatricians in the 1980s there has been an overwhelming increase in the number of the Autistic, creating developmental delays on our children beyond belief. Almost in every state, there has been an increase of autism since the 1980s. In California alone they reported a 273% increase of autistic children since 1987 to 1998, and today that number has risen to over twice the amount.

Today the numbers are staggering in all states.

The medical community and our government knew about the problem in the 1980s when parents started to complain about amoxicillin, but they did nothing about a recall on the drug. Parents were given excuses or assumptions to genetic or environmental factors, but the majority of parents felt that it was not genetics or environmental. It was the new drug, amoxicillin. Moreover, the evidence in my grandbaby's case undoubtedly shows the Amoxicillin Autism Affect is real. This overcomes any hypothetic assumptions.

Fact: Dr. Joan Fallon did a study with 206 autistic children under the age of three years. They were screened by means of a detailed case history. A significant commonality was discerned and that being the level of chronic otitis media. These children were found to have a mean number of 9.96 bouts of otitis media, with a standard error of the mean of +/-1.83. This represents a sum for all 206 children of 2052 bouts of otitis media. These children received a mean number of 12.04 courses of antibiotics, standard error of the mean of +/-.125.

The sum total of courses of antibiotics given to all 206 children was 2480. Of those, 893 courses were Augmentin antibiotic, with 362 of these Augmentin courses administered under the age of one. A propose mechanism whereby the production of clavulanate may yield high levels of urea/ammonia in the child is presented. Further, an examination of this mechanism needs to be undertaken to determine if a subset of children are at risk for neurotoxicity from the use of clavulanic acid in pharmaceutical preparations. Comment in: Med Hypotheses, 2006;66(3):678.

Fact: Amoxicillin/clavulanate (Augmentin) was introduced in 1984 to enhance the activity of Amoxicillin by addition of the beta-lactamase inhibitor, clavulanic acid. During the past years amoxicillin/clavulanate has proven effective for a variety of pediatric infectious diseases, but at the same harming and hurting our children with infectious bacteria build up within the baby's system.

This build up of bacterium will cause problems later for the child as we have been noticing for thirty years to the present. Understand here, our system (the adult) can withstand the danger levels of excessive amoxicillin, but on the baby or the toddler, forget about it! This is the problem here! Pediatricians are over-prescribing Amoxicillin to our children, causing major complications to our children's immune system over an ear infection or any other minor infection.

In many opinions presented by doctors, half the time the patient is misdiagnosed and given over-excessive antibiotics. They have other options less dangerous to the child. It has been proven that taking Amoxicillin will not kill the ear infection, but will kill the pain for a lengthy period of time before the ear infection comes right back. When the ear infection does come back, more regimens of Amoxicillin are given to the child with more return visits to the clinic. In some cases they double the dosage of amoxicillin for management of recurrent and persistent acute otitis media.

This was recommended in 1999 by the Center for Disease Control and Prevention, because of concern about the increased incidence of non-susceptible strains of Streptococcus Pneumonia. My biggest question for the CDC is, "How do you feel now with millions of children being infected with this disease of double dosing amoxicillin for management, causing the amoxicillin autism affect which I believe is true. These doctors in this country prescribing excessive Amoxicillin may or may not realize the alteration it is causing in our children's minds.

Pediatricians are bypassing the danger levels of caution when prescribing medicine to children. It is happening every day! They have no concern whatsoever over how many cycles they gave our babies involving the same medicine since the baby's birth. After all it's o.k. in some cases to double the dose, as the Center for Disease Control recommended. That is crazy! Why is this Amoxicillin a protected antibiotic that is killing and harming our children? Why do they protect it so? In addition, why didn't the CDC step in the 1980s, when an overwhelming number of children were being diagnosed with ASD and Developmental Delay, and parents were claiming autism by the introduction of Amoxicillin. Who are the agencies in this country that can protect our children from diseases if not them? Makes you wonder who or what the CDC, our Medical Community, and our Government Health Department really cares about!

Fact: Doctor James Howenstine - "Excessive antibiotics in children almost certainly stop normal maturation of a healthy immune system (like what happened to my baby). Lack of healthy bacteria in the intestines caused by antibiotics creates an environment in which pieces of partially digested proteins are able to penetrate the barrier of the intestinal lining.

When these abnormal proteins enter the blood, the body properly reacts to them as foreign substances. The foreign proteins cause an antigen antibody reaction producing symptoms and setting the stage for a possible autoimmune illness to develop. This is what happened to my grandbaby's immune system. Dr. J. H. explains that food allergens can also appear, along with impaired absorption of nutrients, which may lead to poor health.

Fact: After 30 years of Amoxicillin since the 1980s, some families today are still convinced that their children are autistic due to Amoxicillin, and the pediatrician does a good job in trying to explain to the parent that is not the case. Pediatricians keep on pushing Amoxicillin for ear infections experienced by babies and children. The reappearance of highly infectious bacteria is caused in part by the overuse and misuse of antibiotics, but the resilience of bacteria also stems from the ingenious biochemistry of the microorganisms themselves.

To survive, microorganisms and fungi mutate into resistant strains. Most Ear Infections Clear Up Without Antibiotics - A newly released report from the Agency for Healthcare Research and Quality (AHRQ) says that children may not always need antibiotics to treat a middle ear infection (otitis media). However, it seems that pediatricians and the medical community refuse to listen to that. Today pediatricians are now confronting bacteria that have built defenses against the use of Amoxicillin with long regimens and excessive treatments of the drug. Question is, do the pediatricians know this?

If pediatricians have knowledge about the defenses bacteria builds up when excessive antibiotics are given, plus the danger level of 20 cycles in a baby's system, then one can only conclude that this is done deliberately or unnoticed on our children. Some infectious bacteria that were once treatable are stronger and often deadly. We have seen many deaths over the years caused by the resistance to Amoxicillin and other antibiotics that no longer work in our children. This, of course, was the reason why my grandbaby's ear infection never went away in spite of the nine months of Amoxicillin, 34 cycles in all that almost killed him in the end.

Fact: Dr. Hendley: Americans are becoming more and more de-sensitized to the effects of antibiotics because they have been over medicated on these drugs. Thus, when they are infected with bacterium, the Amoxicillin and other antibiotics are infected. Dr. Owen Hendley wrote in the Oct. 10. 2002 edition of the New England Journal of Medicine, those Placebo-controlled trials found that ear infections disappeared in one week in 81 percent of Placebo recipients, compared with 94 percent of antibiotic recipients.

In most cases within the survey of 1 in 100, these children had over twenty cycles of Amoxicillin in their first three to five years to be diagnosed with ADD, DD, and Autism & ADHD. Many good doctors in this country who care about our children's immune system, their digestive tract, and their development, urge that pediatricians avoid the over-prescription of Amoxicillin and other antibiotics.

If the medical community would have taken time to listen to the parents in the 1980s, maybe they would have listened to Dr. Hendley, instead of using Amoxicillin. They could have re-entered the old cures. My grandbaby would have not had an ear infection for nine months, and his mind would have not been compromised for life, without the destruction from Amoxicillin. I believe that if the baby's doctors would have treated my grandbaby with the placebo treatment from the 1980s or any other option other than Amoxicillin, I would not be here crying my heart out, and writing to the world about my baby's torture that almost killed him with nine months of Amoxicillin, with me at the helm obeying doctors' orders to hurt my baby. Excuse my anger but I am very upset at this country's government for allowing this to happen to my baby, and all the other families' children over the years.

Moreover, for what? Money, profit, gain of control, the stock market? Why? Can you tell me why, Mr. President? Why? These are just a handful of facts to prove that the Amoxicillin Autism Affect is real and alive. You the people, your families, you must put your foot down to explain to our pediatricians in a nice way and prevent Pharmaceutical companies from hurting our babies and our children, prescribing drugs that are harmful in altering our children's system and minds!

Prescribing Amoxicillin over excessively past the duration period, and over 20 cycles of Amoxicillin in the first 12 years of the child's life are killing our children, and causing them Autism Developmental Delay Disorder. Interfering with our babies' immune system all in the name of Money, Power and Greed, must stop! There is not enough paper to write down how many children have died or have been compromised as a result of this recipe of amoxicillin. Many families do not know that their children have a disorder. Instead, they think it is a disciplinary problem that the child has. Doctors and researchers have been arguing with the medical community over this destruction to our children here in America for decades. Do you think me and all families who feel like I do are crazy? We really have to worry about keeping our children out of harm's way. Pediatricians, who took that sacred oath for healing the sick and for our children, should keep that oath in their hearts.

Instead, we see them drowning our children with Amoxicillin, which has a record of harming children internally with permanent damage. New laws and regulations that protect these doctors from over excessive medicating is a result of Mr. George Bush pushing and passing these laws against malpractice cases of these kinds. That is why many grossly negligent doctors are still in practice. Many of us parents have children who fell to the Amoxicillin Experiments over the years—experiments that have injured our children for life internally.

We are caring law-abiding citizens who follow the law, and the new law has a bite on capping penalties when it comes to malpractice. Thus, now 10 out of 10 attorneys will not touch a malpractice case unless you have money to invest, because they would not touch the case on pro-bono. The only way to start the recovery process of 1 in 88 children being diagnosed with autism, is to put an end to Amoxicillin for children and babies, and bring back the placebo recipients or another option other than Amoxicillin.

Start listening to these great doctors and researchers who have told the medical community, time after time, after time, to stop the excessive Amoxicillin and other antibiotic treatments, which do not work on ear infections. Stop the Amoxicillin Experiments. In addition, for all doctors, if you want or need a place to start in helping our children, start by not prescribing Amoxicillin to our children. Give our children another option, or better yet, make a new drug that will be harmless to our children.

In addition, start listing the doctors who are against the Amoxicillin for the good of our children here in America. Let us get back that caring heart from the good old days. Let us start caring for these children's future for the long run. Stop paying blood money by making that infant or child returns to your clinic over and over for as long as possible. Wake up to what you are doing to these children. You can't blame me for the way I feel and what I've learned, so wake up, pediatricians, and remember that you're a doctor for the children first, or did you forget?

8
ANTIBIOTIC BRIEF

Another brief was written up by Terry A. Rondberg, D.C. called "Under the Influence of Modern Medicine." For me this is another piece of research that has been ignored by the medical community. If the medical community had paid attention to that brief sixteen years ago, we would have saved millions of children from Autism Spectrum Disorder by this time.

These harmful bacteria have even killed many children. Amoxicillin has not only destroyed immune systems and the child's intestines and caused developmental problems for our children for years, it also causes over 400 child deaths each year in America.

When antibiotics were first developed they were considered a "miracle drug" because they seemed to be able to aid the body in fighting off infections and invading bacteria, but they came at a deadly price for our children. The drug actually was helpful for some people with weakened immune systems who needed outside intervention to get through immediate and acute health crises. However, this miracle drug started to be abused. Even a miracle drug can be abused, and it's an abuse of a medical drug that will go down in history along with your everyday street drugs. Medical doctors, thinking in their minds that they must have a cure for everything, started prescribing the drug after nearly every office visit. Even for conditions that could not be helped at all by antibiotics, they still prescribed the drug. At the same time, they were compromising their patients—the infants' and children's immune system.

They pumped the drug into their systems and now decades later, we are paying the price with antibiotic-resistant super-bacteria and impaired natural antibody functions. Tragically, despite warnings from the **World Health Organization**, and from more progressive health care experts, medical doctors and pediatricians still rely on the drug, especially the #1 antibiotic, Amoxicillin, that is used on babies and children. The World Health Organization warns that the spread of many devastating diseases may be blamed on the overuse of antibiotics throughout the world.

Each year hundreds of thousands of children die worldwide because of this dilemma with Amoxicillin. The optimism of a relatively few years ago that many of these diseases could be brought under control, has led to a fatal complacency. This complacency is now costing millions of lives. Do you think your government cares about that? I do not think so! The World Health Organization also reports and lists several other critical factors including poverty and overcrowding, and they single out - *the uncontrolled and inappropriate use of antibiotics,* as one of the primary reasons for the outbreak of drug-resistant strains of infectious diseases. The antibiotics are misused to treat the wrong kind of infections, and the wrong dosage (Over excessive). The overuse of antibiotics has been shown many times to weaken the body's natural immune system (as in what happened to Christopher). Amoxicillin and other antibiotics are frequently used to prevent middle ear infections that affect millions of children in America each year.

However, a study supported by the **Agency for Health Care Policy and Research** indicated that the use of these antibiotics is not a good idea for ear infections, it is only marginally effective and the infection will return. The study showed that children with recurrent middle ear infections, - that is three infections within six months or four in a year, - fare about the same as children given a placebo, with 61-64% remaining free of new infections during the study period.

This shows that a placebo has been replaced with an antibiotic has no business being used for ear infections on children. Researchers say that the excessive antibiotic use, which has the potential to promote acquisition of antibiotic-resistant bacterial pneumonia already, is becoming more prevalent as the years go by. A scientific literature review published in the New England Journal of Medicine has added more dangers to the overuse and misuse of antibiotics. They explained in a research project, "It was soon evident that bacterial pathogens were unlikely to surrender unconditionally, because some pathogens rapidly became resistant to many of the first effective drugs. Each time the bacteria becomes resistant to the existing antibiotic, the response has been to develop a new one." In essence, the medical profession through its use of antibiotics has bred numerous "super bacteria" which are resistant to many of the current antibiotics. The adaptability of the bacteria makes it nearly impossible to create drugs that will stop them. This is what is going on with Amoxicillin and ear infections on babies and children, a build up of resistance that is leading doctors in this country to overuse Amoxicillin 7 to 10 days for starters.

I believe they do this just to prove something that may be fatal to the child. In fact, new drugs are more likely to breed even stronger bacteria that are more resilient. Most infants are given antibiotics during the first six months despite repeated warnings about the overuse and misuse of antibiotics. What happened to my grandbaby with the 9 months of Amoxicillin started at 6 months of age, but I did not know any better back then, which is something I have to live with for the rest of my life.

However, today I know everything I need to know. Doctors in this country continue to pump the drugs into our nation's children at an alarming rate. Another medical study by these great doctors who care for our children showed 70% of all infants in the United States are subjected to their first course of antibiotics during the first 200 days of their lives. Researchers found that otitis media (middle ear infection) was the most common reason for antibiotic treatment in infants and Amoxicillin is the most common antibiotic prescribed. In recent years more and more health care professionals again, have warned the medical community that the misuse of antibiotics as a line of first defense has not only weakened the natural immune system, but created a variety of super bacteria which are resistant to any antibiotics. It is incredible to think that in this country of freedom and free will, the richest country in the world would allow this horrible attack of ASD & DD to reach our children through Amoxicillin.

What's more incredible is allowing it with the knowledge that not all pediatricians will heed to the warnings of top studies on the antibiotic's destruction of our infants and children's immune system, which causes the Amoxicillin Autism Affect. Most of us that fell victims to the destruction of our babies in autism feel hopeless and disgusted, but I am here to tell you that two wrongs don't make a right. Start writing to the President and tell him the reason you are writing to him.

Even if it seems that nothing will happen if you write letters, still write them. Tell them that over excessive Amoxicillin for our children is unacceptable. I wrote to my governor and almost every official in Florida and all of them told me that the doctors that put my baby in the hospital did nothing wrong. Their protection of the doctors, and the Amoxicillin that is destroying our children's health, shows all Floridians that our government does not care to hear about your family's problems. When it comes to Amoxicillin and the danger levels that have caused your baby major medical problems, the governor should be the first one at the plate. Sometimes I feel like I live in another country. Our government does whatever they feel like even if it goes against the people.

Our government never listens to the people. Our government allows harm to reach our children. As far as I can see, all corruption that is going against our children's health with Amoxicillin is because of the drive for money and power, profits and gain for the investors of antibiotics, and the pharmaceutical companies, and our government lobbyists.

In addition, with all the corruption that is going on in medicine and medical doctors we have in the industry, I can say that the people we vote into office to run this country say things that we want to hear, and in the end can you hear the laughter? We are their suckers. How much more pain and misery must our children suffer? When are we going to smell the coffee and wake up? These pharmaceutical companies and doctors, who follows the road of greed in this country, are killing our children slowly. Something to stop thinking about, and do something about it! This is all evidence that is hard to deny about the Amoxicillin Autism Affect that has been with us for 30 years. It is hard to deny the facts I am presenting you right here, right now.

9
THE AMOXICILLIN DIAGNOSIS

Now, let's look at the real diagnosis of amoxicillin besides killing infections. The baby was discharged in September 23, 2005 from the hospital, a few weeks after we had the ear tubes put in. After that, we decided to wait a few months before we had him tested for his development because we felt that he was not ready after all the misery and pain he had been through.

We had Christopher eating yogurts to build up his immune system, along with the proper diet that coincides with building his system back to a functioning level. We could see his behavior is different, that of confusion. This, of course, would take some time before we could see some improvements in his system, as we were told from the hospital.

In December, 2005, we had him retested at Early Steps Children's Medical Services, and it was from this testing that I came to realize that indeed my baby would be in trouble for the rest of his life. The testing concluded that he was two years developmentally delayed in all his motor skills, and on all other fronts. They explained that eventually the baby would reach a level to be able to learn certain things, but that we had major work ahead. My grandbaby does not speak a word now, but eventually will speak. As time passes, he will not be 100% as he should be. Instead, in time, we may see improvement with hard work around the clock from us, and he may need special schooling and instructions. We were told that the change in behavior and speech would not come easy, but instead his behavior and speech would falter as time passes, because of his new way of life in being Developmentally Delayed. My wife and I started to cry after the evaluation.

I quickly asked the Occupational Therapist another question - How is it that we had the baby tested when he was 9 months old and he passed his evaluation, and today, at 18 months old, he is autism delayed? 'You are telling us that he is about two years behind just because he cannot speak, or do potty, and maybe he fades out into the twilight and he does not play patty cake. Aren't these things normal for a child? They replied indeed. They confirmed that the doctors at All Children Hospital were correct in telling us about our baby's future.

She looked at me with regret and explained to me that this is happening every day to many of our children in America, and the reason, she says, is that nobody knows why? She agreed with me that it is not normal for a child to be developmentally delayed after the child has been tested nine months earlier with a passing mark. Then she told us, in my grandbaby's case it just may be because of the nine months of Amoxicillin in his system, that this may have occurred, but she can't say for sure because her expertise is not in that area. That is when I finally absorbed and took everything in - that indeed the emergency room doctors at the hospital were right about the Amoxicillin and my baby's future. The examiner told us that the baby would need speech therapy, occupational therapy, and developmental therapy. That being said from a Licensed Occupational Therapist of Early Steps, they gave me the will to do some in-depth research on my own regarding all the diagnoses that were declared on the baby at the hospital. I prepared myself for a long struggle and an uphill battle in researching the complications that lay ahead for me, while taking care of my family at the same time.

As time passed, my baby could never speak or do certain things with his hands. I was doing my research around the clock. While I was doing my research every day, my tears were coming down my face at the same time because of what I was learning on all the suffering that children are going through in this country—even death at the hands of medical doctors. One month later January, 2006, I decided to get a second opinion and took Christopher to All Children's Hospital for another evaluation.

Dr. Shapiro, a Developmental Specialist, concluded his diagnosis, and found that "yes" Christopher was Developmentally Delayed. This, of course, proved conclusively that the Occupational Therapist of Early Steps was correct. I fell into a world of anger and I started to continue my research on Autism and Developmental Delay cases. What I found out was more depressing regarding how children get to be this way. I have to say that there is not enough paper in the world to write the enormous amount of information the public needs to know on this subject. I have to let the world know what is going on here somehow, someway. I have to be brief with the most important information families need to know to protect their babies and children. In my opinion it is a well-corrupted operation that is going on in this country, using our children for profits, starting with our own government allowing this destruction on our children.

To think that a baby is born not for the purpose that God has for that child, but for the greed of mankind. So let me be brief, these are the damages that Amoxicillin did to my baby's system that landed him in the hospital almost dead. Just another case caused by amoxicillin on my grandbaby, only this time it's different.

Diagnosis of Baby Christopher:

<u>Diagnosis # (1)</u> - Acute Gastroenteritis - Acute Gastroenteritis is a serious health issue and is responsible for over five hundred thousand hospitalizations of children in the United States each year. It is a long and potentially lethal bout of stomach flu, with the majority of cases caused by Amoxicillin and other antibiotics. After having 34 cycles of Amoxicillin for nine months in baby Christopher's system, this caused the bloody acid diarrhea that he suffered on his last leg of life. It inflamed the gastrointestinal tract causing the Acute Gastroenteritis. Other causes of acute gastroenteritis are bacterial infection and viruses, which my grandbaby had developed during the nine months of Amoxicillin. This type of gastroenteritis has caused the death of many, and if treated on time may be subdued but with later complications, depending on the destruction that has occurred within the baby's system. Although there are other methods of transmission of acute gastroenteritis, we have ruled out all possibilities. Amoxicillin is the #1 drug that causes many complications for babies and children if the drug is misused.

In this case it's obvious because of the bloody acid diarrhea, those bacteria and viruses were shutting down my grandbaby's body during the nine-month period. We have children dying each year around the world, even in this country of Acute Gastroenteritis. We have 300 to 400 deaths each year in the United States due to this problem. The numbers may not be as high as developing countries, but are overwhelming to say the least.

Makes you wonder why the news media does not talk about it much. Overall, 6 million children die each year of Infectious Gastroenteritis from Acute Gastroenteritis.

One death of an infant or child in this country of Acute Gastroenteritis is more than enough. For me, the 300 to 400 that die each year in this country of Acute Gastroenteritis can be prevented by eliminating the source of action. Amoxicillin for children must be pulled to the sideline.

Diagnosis # (2) - Chronic Otitis Media - Chronic Otitis Media (COM) is the term used to describe a variety of signs, symptoms, and physical findings that result from long term damage to the middle ear by infection and inflammation. Christopher began his ear infection when he was 6 months old and continued to have the ear infection for 9 months, treated with Amoxicillin that put him in the hospital.

After doing my research I was shocked to learn that until recently, nearly every American child with an ear infection who visited a doctor received antibiotics, starting with the #1 Amoxicillin drug of choice for our children. In one region of the U.S. more than 75% of children received the Amoxicillin before they were 7 months old, (Just like my grandbaby) and the most common reason for this medication was acute otitis media, But the irony of this is that the Amoxicillin does not work in killing the infection in the ear. All it does is take the pain away.

A chronic ear infection is more destructive than an acute ear infection because the effects are prolonged or repeated. It may cause permanent damage to the ear and induce developmental issues if the ear infection continues for months on end. Major studies now indicate (now when the medical community is finally coming out with some truth on the subject), that antibiotics are unnecessary in the majority of cases of ear infections. Between 80 % and 90 % of all children with uncomplicated ear infections recover within a week without antibiotics.

The purpose of antibiotics is to kill harmful bacteria, and otitis media means middle ear inflammation - not necessarily bacterial infection. Amoxicillin has been shown to increase the likelihood of repeated ear infections, as in the case of my grandbaby. One reason is, when a pediatrician prescribes Amoxicillin, the underlying cause of the ear infection is usually ignored and left untreated.

Example - Streptococcus pneumonias, also known as pneumococcus is commonly found in the nose and throat. This bacterium is responsible for many cases of ear infections, which is why the antibiotics are prescribed. However, your child can have pneumococcus and not be sick. It will only cause trouble if it is trapped in the middle ear. Once trapped, the bacteria can and will reproduce rapidly and become an infection. Experts and some great doctors in this field have been saying what the medical community refuses to listen.

They recommend that if you must give your baby or child Amoxicillin, the duration period should only be 10 days for children under 6 years old. If the antibiotic does not work during that period, the pediatrician should go after other options available for the child, and they know what options are available. They gave my baby 9 months of Amoxicillin, 34 cycles in all, a high rate of antibiotic resistance that was not killing the infection but landing him in the hospital almost dead, and the doctors got away with it. Or did they?

Diagnosis # (3) C-Difficile Bacteria - C- Difficile also known by its name Clostridium Difficile is a bacterium that causes a serious case of acid watery diarrhea and more serious intestinal conditions such as colitis. It is lethal if not treated on time, especially on infants and children, it could lead to death. It is responsible for thousands of deaths each year here in the U.S. and internationally. It is very contagious and hospitalization treatment would be needed.

The medical community would say that C-Difficile is best known to attack the body through hospitals or a long-term care facility, which is true, but C- Difficile is not confined exclusively to hospitals and care facilities; it is everywhere - in the soil, air, water, human and animal feces and on most surfaces. The bacteria do not create problems until they grow in abnormally large numbers in the intestinal tract of people taking antibiotics or other anti-microbial drugs.

My baby's intestinal tract was in ruins with C-Diffcile, and lethal for a baby at 15 months old. Antibiotics can cause harmful bacteria to proliferate in the intestine. It is also well known by the medical community here in this country, and among all pediatricians who care for your babies, that the # 1 antibiotic for pediatricians Amoxicillin is the most implicated in C-Difficile infections.

Also implicated are Ampicillin, Clindamycin, Fluoroquinolones, and Cephalosporin in C-Difficile infections. Senior citizens are also victims of this infection caused by too many antibiotics administered for a lengthy duration, leading some elderly to their death. Your intestinal tract contains hundreds of kinds of bacteria (Intestinal Flora). However, many bacteria in the intestinal tract are essential, helping to synthesize certain vitamins and stimulating the immune system, but with the interference of an over load of Amoxicillin building infectious bacteria in the intestinal tract; this will disrupt the good bacteria that the body needs.

These bacteria are the good bacteria that our body needs, because some play a key role in suppressing the growth of harmful organisms. However, when you take an antibiotic to treat an infection, especially when you're taking excessive antibiotics over the long period like they did to my grandbaby; it will destroy these beneficial bacteria as well as the bacteria that is causing your illness.

Without enough healthy bacteria in your system, dangerous pathogens such as C-Difficile will quickly grow out of control and cause serious damage in your intestinal tract and your immune system. It is especially dangerous for a baby's immune system to be disrupted and the damage occurs a hundred times quicker than on an adult. This is a recipe for developmental problems as years pass if the baby lives through it at all. This subject on C-Difficile bacteria is long and extensive. Believe me when I tell you that if you or your baby is infected with this bacterium, rest assured that your doctor or your pediatrician will not say it came from excessive amoxicillin. They will protect their reputation and protect the antibiotics that they prescribed for your baby. Each year over 2500 die in Canada over C-Difficile. Over 6000 die in British hospitals. In the U.S. over 400.000 are hospitalized each year, and over 500 die of diarrhea related illness with C-Difficile bacteria. The numbers of dead among children are getting higher each year because of these bacteria. Something to think about.

<u>Diagnosis # (3A)</u> C-Difficile Toxin B (+) - Is more potent than toxin A in damaging human colonic epithelium in vitro. The colon is 10 times more sensitive to damaging effects of toxin B than toxin A, suggesting that toxin B is more important than toxin A in the pathogenesis of C-Difficile Colitis in man - Imagine this in a baby or a child. An overload of Amoxicillin is given to babies and children based on a theory that by giving the child antibiotic over the duration must be continued because the infection did not go away after a couple of cycles. But it is not sensible.

It is crazy to try to prove to parents that Amoxicillin will work if it doesn't work on the duration period the first time. For any doctor to try to look good to the parents by doing this is the most idiotic thing you can do as a professional doctor. When antibiotics are given to children, especially babies, the micro flora in the large intestine change and this allows rapid proliferation of C-Difficile. That begins to release toxins in the intestine. The toxins can get through the intestinal lining and spread to the rest of the body, producing toxemia. C- Difficile produces two types of toxins that cause diarrhea.

Toxin (A) - Causes inflammation and secretion of fluids in the large intestine, but toxin (B) is 1.000 times more potent and causes severe damage to the mucosal lining of the intestine that will produce blood in the feces. This is what happened to my grandbaby.

This is the torture that my baby went through in the hands of not one - but four pediatricians. How crazy is that, my baby almost died! What are you doctors thinking when you do something like this to innocent children? Shame on all you doctors who have been doing this to our children for 30 years with this crazy antibiotic, Amoxicillin. This must stop! This will stop one way or another! Do you hear me! Do you hear me, Mr. President of the United States of America - Save Our Children from This ever Growing Problem!

Diagnosis # (4) Rotavirus AGE - Rotavirus is a viral infection among young children. It is the most common cause of diarrhea in U.S. children with a growing number of deaths along the way. The diarrhea turns to a watery dark green acid, but in my baby's case, he had blood in his diarrhea and even in his eyes. After three years, my grandbaby's stool is still green in color, but not in diarrhea form. Instead over the years it has been pasty with no blood, and would remain green on occasions for a very long time, that is, for many years. The doctors told us at All Children that the baby was going to have the green stool for quite some time because of the destruction in the baby's system. Rotavirus is a leading cause of death among children in third world countries. Worldwide, over 10 million children die from this each year. These countries do not have access to clean water supplies and IV fluids for proper hospitalization treatments. In the United States over 200 children die each year from Rotavirus, with the leading cause the excessive use of Amoxicillin in the child's system that causes the diarrhea, that causes the Rotavirus.

The virus works by attacking the lining of the small intestine causing often-copious loss of fluids and electrolytes, as in the case of my grandbaby. The biggest danger with this illness is dehydration. Signs of severe dehydration include irritability, lethargy, sunken eyes, sunken soft spots in infants, dry mouth and tongue, less frequent bathroom trips and dry diapers for more than a couple of hours. If you notice these signs, it is imperative that you contact your physician immediately.

I suggest that you take your baby to an emergency room ASAP—then contact the baby's pediatrician afterwards. When your baby is hospitalized, intravenous rehydration is usually given and will save your baby's life. Treatment at home includes plenty of rest and use of an oral electrolyte replacement solution such as Pedialyte or Gatorade according to pediatricians' recommendation. I would think twice about Gatorade with the high amounts of sugar that can further irritate the intestinal tract. Begin giving Pedialyte at the first sign of loose stools and vomiting. Electrolyte is a medical term for salts, specifically ions. The term electrolyte means that this ion is electrically charged and moves to either a negative (cathode) or positive (anode) electrode. Electrolytes are important because they are what your cells use to maintain voltage across their cell membranes and to carry electrical impulses (nerve impulses & muscle contractions) across themselves and to other cells.

Your kidneys work to keep the electrolyte concentrations in your blood constant despite changes in your body. These electrolytes must be replaced to keep the electrolyte concentrations of your body fluids constant. Therefore, these are all the diagnoses that my baby had when he landed in the hospital almost dead. And to think, on that last week of his dying days before we landed him in the hospital, the pediatricians that were taking care of him at the time refused to put our baby in the hospital, because they felt that my grandbaby at the time did not need to go to the hospital.

They prescribed all 9 months of Amoxicillin, so what does that say about these pediatricians practicing medicine in this country? It breaks my heart knowing the torture that my baby's system was put through, and the mere fact that I was not knowledgeable at the time, and now it's up to me to try to fix his system as much as possible through tough love and early intervention. The year 2006 would prove to be very challenging in the efforts for grandbaby, and the start of a long-term challenge for us, his grandparents. Let us look at how important early intervention is for your child and mine…………..

10
EARLY INTERVENTION A MUST!

In January, 2006, we went to the baby's new pediatrician, Dr. Gambia, after we found out from All Children's Hospital that the baby was Developmentally Delayed. We told Dr. Gambia about the baby's diagnosis by All Children, and Early Steps Children's Medical Services. We asked her if she had any input for us. Surprisingly, she told us that the baby was too young yet at 19 ½ months, even after we told her about the diagnosis from the hospital.

This is how some pediatricians think, which is wrong. She told me for the moment, after what the baby been through, not to put the baby on an active intervention program. She said we should wait until the baby is at least 3 or 4 years old. She says that children have their own time when to break out of silence, or exert their motor skills.

Of course, we looked at her as if she was crazy, but not surprised because this is a small town where all doctors know each other, and we are sure that this new pediatrician knows the doctors in town who almost killed our baby. Therefore, for now we would play along with this new pediatrician, and make our own decisions along the way. She does not know that we are already going to early intervention for our baby through Early Steps. After doing some research I find that there are many doctors in this country who feel you should wait until the baby is much older for early intervention, and a minority will tell you to go ahead at 18 months. We started to have our baby evaluated at 9 months of age because of all the Amoxicillin entering his body, before he landed in the emergency room. I guess this Dr. Gambia thinks in her mind that she has all the right answers, as do most pediatricians. I say the earliest as possible have the baby tested.

It is so important for you as a parent to realize that you are the decision maker for your baby's health, not your baby's doctor. Your baby's doctor is there to tell you what he or she believes are best for your baby's healthcare. If you ever see a red flag popping up, then it's time for you to question the doctor and make the final decision for the safety of your child. I know some families in the town where I live in my opinion their children of ages three to fives, needed to be evaluated for some type of disorder. The signs where there.

These are good families with caring hearts, after I spotted the signs a few red flags in the children's speech and behavior patterns. I made contact and educated them on what I see. You may have seen the same thing among your families and friends, and I know that some of you will not approach your friends or even acquaintances to share the thought that maybe their child needs a little testing. I believe as part of being a good person in the eyes of God that it is your responsibility to make that parent realize that they are passing up something very important for their child's development. The way you would communicate that message is to compliment those families on their child's ability to learn; remember all children are learnable. Do not be afraid of reaching out to help a child even if the parent throws a negative left hook at your jaw. Believe me, later on when you're not looking, that parent will smack her cheek in appreciation. The parents I ran into refused to have their children tested, because their pediatrician felt that they are just kids who are growing.

Some children take a little longer than other kids. Some may to do certain things that kids normally do at their age. These are the excuses that some parents are giving me. Of course, I felt hurt when they told me that, but I did my job as a good person. There are a lot of good doctors and pediatricians in this country; I know this. However, we must decide what is best of our children's lives, and not put all our trust in doctors. Some families I spoke with would rather listen to their doctor than their spouse.

A doctor's opinion should be observed and examined first before you follow it, after exhausting all other possibilities you can muster in your mind. This action on your part is in no means, and in no way disrespectful nor trying to be smarter than these doctors are. These doctors are intelligent people and I am sure they know what time it is. There is always a handful in the bunch that make the news on bad judgment calls when it comes to a child, and that judgment call would have affected your child's life, right or wrong.

Remember this is your child's healthcare and it is not a two-way street, it is only one-way, your way, your child, your house. This action on your part of being more vigilant and stronger with questions for your pediatrician about your baby's healthcare, is not personal. It's just protecting your child from some doctors who hurt children that we hear about every now and then—stories like this one that happened to my baby. It has not been an easy road for me and my wife since the baby was six months old.

In addition, the sacrifices that we make and have to apply for these children, will cross the line of sanity at times for us, because it is a hard task. I know it's hard sometimes because you have to deal with the child's meltdowns, and when he has them in public, it could be at the store, or at the school, and, of course, in the house all the time. This is the adjustment that we parents have to make for ourselves, and at the same time we have to educate those around us and our child, so people can understand what a special needs child is all about.

In your home, you have to be very understanding with your child who has developmental delay or autism spectrum disorder, because these children do not understand right from wrong like the normal child does. The wires in their brain are not quite connected like the normal child. Their neurotransmitters have been compromised.

It could be the child was born with Autism or DD genetically, or it could be they received the disorder from a long-term destructive regiment of antibiotics. The fact is that we parents have to educate ourselves, and we have to find a way to communicate to the child what is right and what is wrong using constructive techniques. Remember this will take years before you have your child at a level of comfort for learning and communicating in society, but you have to start now.

These children always want to be rewarded because they know in their minds that something is not right with them, so they try so hard to please you, so you can accept them by rewarding them. When they see themselves among other children they want to feel accepted, loved, and wanted, but they do not know how to go about it. The feeling of love and comfort is want they understand more than anything else. You carried them for nine months in your belly with comfort and love.

With a normal child, every now and then a parent may think that a child needs a hand on his hinny, even if it draws a tear or a little scream behind it, because you know that child understands, and just wants to be difficult. I have to say to you that five fingers on his little hinny is not the answer for any child, unless you want to go to jail. Being gentle and speaking low tone even if you have a screamer, will show much more success than what's happening now. If you have a teenager or adult autism, constructive explanations should be before any yelling. Being this way will help shape any child or adult with autism from making wrong choices, you do not have to be confuse or physical, because in the end you loose, and so does your child. With a child that has Autism Spectrum Disorder and Developmental Delay, giving him a little spanking would be crazy. There's no telling what would happen to your child's mind set, and you may loose him more than one way.

For one thing, you will trigger his meltdowns and confuse him as to what he did he wrong. Even if you explain it to him that he did wrong, he will not understand and start building on anger and yelling out what he sees and hears. Instead of spanking him – If you must by way of your beliefs, you can sit him down on a chair for a few, until he calms down, then speak to him gently This works better on developmentally delayed children and autistic children with slow communication. They understand this type of time-out, better than a spanking that the normal child understands right from wrong. Sit him down a chair where he is not allowed to get up, this will be his thinking chair.

Believe me when I say that he will understand something's with sitting him down, and he wants to be free to do things. Do not give in to anything that you feel that your child wants if it's wrong for the child's behavior pattern. For better communication, you should try to go down to his level, in character of course, and just maybe you can grab his attention at a level of understanding and communication. Remember, as your baby grows older at two years old, at three years old, at four years of age, no matter what type of disorder whether it be Autism Spectrum Disorder or any other type of disorder, these children are learnable if you take the time for them. In addition, I find that these children can be taught decency, respect, and politeness at the earliest year possible. You must work harder with these children between the ages of one and five years old. If you suspect something is wrong and the baby is not doing what he or she is supposed to be doing between these ages, look for the red flags, be more constructive with your child.

Remember your children did not ask to come to this world; we put them here. I am tired of hearing that some parents hit their special needy children for any little reason, because the parent is so overwhelmed. If that is the case, the parent can seek some relief by attending classes and discussion groups that can help. There is so much to learn on this subject because everyday a new idea is formed for the educational production for these children, and you are the inventor —the parents and grandparents.

A parent's sacrifice to learn techniques and skills that work for the children with these disorders is what they expect from you. The parent is the child's only prayer that he has for survival in this complicated world. For these children the parent is the teacher and the doctor with a binding love and security. This is why we as parents must sacrifice every moment we can muster for them - because we love them, and we want the best for our children. When you are at the store, you have to develop a relationship between the children and the stores you visit.

If the meltdowns are too much at the stores for you to handle, create a deterrent like a reading book with pictures of his favorite characters. It is important if you are going out with the children to try to make it as comfortable as possible. You know he or she is only 3 or 5 years old, and at this age, they are going to want something from the store one way or another, and if mommy hits them, they will just cry louder.

We have to be ready at all times with an idea for the child, in order to grab the child's attention or have him doing something that is fun for him. However, unbelievably, if nothing else works, and you've tried everything in the pot, try a little surprise. Give them something while you shop such as a cookie so they will entertain themselves. At first, it will be simple, and you will know the things he likes, but when things start to change a little and he wants more than you are giving him, use a little bribe with the things he likes. Believe me, it works.

We have to create surprises for them sometimes, and then gradually you can explain what is right or wrong, so he can do it, and understand the right or the wrong. Even though sometimes surprises can be costly, it's the language they understand. We have to remember in regard to children with disorders, the neurotransmitters are not quite doing their jobs in their brains, like yours and mine. Their development have been compromised, and we have to bear in mind that we somehow have to try and put the pieces together for them, whatever it takes. God will love you for stepping up to the plate, and so will your children. I cannot stress enough the importance of having your baby tested at an early age—as early as six to ten months old, and start from there. The earlier you look into your child's development, the more at ease you will feel. Again, if your pediatrician feels it's too early to have the baby tested, that is just her opinion. It's o.k. to go ahead and make an appointment to your local Early Steps Children's Medical Services.

I did not follow my baby's Pediatrician Gambia's advice about waiting until he was three or four years old to test my grandbaby, to find out if what I suspected was happening to my grandson or not. That's crazy! However, I was stupid enough to follow the recommendations of the four pediatricians that took care of my grandson's health and almost killed him, without making a proper judgment call when it came to my grandson, so he landed in the hospital almost dead.

I followed all instructions of these doctors to the letter, and put all my trust in them instead of thinking twice. Look where it got me, look where it got my grandbaby! I was stupid back then by not knowing anything about the drugs these doctors were making me feed my grandbaby. I did not know anything about Amoxicillin - But today I do!

Now, you too know a lot more about Amoxicillin you give to your babies because you are reading this book, and that is good. I would hope you will take precautions when it comes to Amoxicillin for your baby, for ear infections or other ailments. If you do these things for the safety of your baby, you will see your baby grow the way you expected your baby to grow, and that is a beautiful thing for your baby and you. If at the moment you are experiencing something like what my grandbaby went through, and your baby has been on Amoxicillin for weeks on end over an ear infection that just doesn't want to go away, contact the nearest All Children's Hospital in your area.

If you do not have one in your area, take your baby right now to the nearest Emergency Room Hospital without your baby's pediatrician's permission, as I did. That is how we saved our baby's life. You need to recognize your child's growth and development steps, from birth until he is 5 years old, these are the most critical years for the baby. Those years are the important years, to see if the child is developing properly to the norm with their motor skills, communication skills and so on. Do not let those years go by without you yourself giving your child observations along the way.

In addition, if your child is older than three years old, it's never too late for observation, and motor skill testing, and communication testing. Test them for everything. There are many Children's Medical Services in which you can call and make an appointment. However, I will share with you the first critical three years of indicators that you can look for. Babies and toddlers grow and develop at their own pace, but usually can do the following activities by the age of three. I will describe to you some of the key things to look for. If you can spot a problem, then please check with your pediatricians, or contact your local Early Steps Children Medical Center and draw your concerns of what the baby should be doing up to 36 months old.

THREE MONTHS OLD: TYPICAL ACTIVITIES:
* Pushes up head and chest when on tummy.
* Moves body actively in response to voice.
* Chuckles, coos
* Enjoys touch.
* Turns head toward sounds.
* Soothes with cuddling
* Smiles.
* Watches faces and objects.
* Kicks feet, moves hands.
* Brings hands to mouth.

Indicators for concern at three months
    ** Does not watch moving objects.
    ** Does not startle at sounds.

SIX MONTHS OLD: TYPICAL ACTIVITIES.
* Rolls from stomach to back.
* Has good head control.
* Laughs while playing.
* Reaches and grasps toys, objects.
* Has predictable sleep pattern.

* Moves objects from Hand to hand.
* Sits, but may need support.
* Babbles more than two sounds.

Indicators for concern at 6 months
   ** Unable to roll over.
   ** Difficulty lifting head.
   ** Does not turn head to direction of sound.

NINE MONTHS OLD: TYPICAL ACTIVITIES.
* Looks for hidden toys.
* Throws toys or objects.
* Pulls self up, stands while holding on
* Feeds self finger foods such as cereal.
* Imitates sounds like "ooh" and "ahh"

Indicators for concern at 9 months.
   ** Unable to sit by self.
   ** Difficulty picking up Objects.
   ** Not imitating or babbling

TWELVE MONTHS OLD: TYPICAL ACTIVITIES.
* Pulls self up and stands.
* Says "Mama", "Baba", and "Dada".
* Begins to follow simple directions. (Please come here, drink your milk)
* Waves goodbye.
* Presses buttons on phone, toys.
* Enjoys being read to.

Indicators for concerns at 12 months
   ** Does not use single words like "Mama" or "Dada".
   ** Difficulty crawling.
   ** Needs to Use hand to maintain sitting.

FIFTEEN MONTHS OLD: TYPICAL ACTIVITIES

* Stands or steps towards or walks.

* Knows or says 4 or 5 words.

* Helps to dress by holding out arms or legs.

* Curious - will explore on own.

Indicators for concerns at 15 months
- ** Unable to stand-alone.
- ** Does not point to objects, people.
- ** Does not hold up cup.

EIGHTEEN MONTHS OLD: TYPICAL ACTIVITIES.

* Walks well, runs a little.

* Scribbles

* Prefers to feed self.

* Knows names of things, people.

* Plays alongside of other children.

* Squats to pick up toy.

* Beginning pretend play.

Indicators for concerns at 18 months
- ** Unable to walk without help.
- ** Does not Say at least 15 words.
- ** Not able to feed self with spoon.

TWENTY-FOUR MONTHS OLD: TYPICAL ACTIVITIES.

* Kicks large balls.

* Recognizes familiar pictures, books.

* Engages in pretend play (using spoon as an airplane)

* Uses 2 or 3 words together.

* Says "mine"

* Jumps in place.

Indicators for concerns at 24 months:
- ** Does not follow simple directions.
- ** Does not pretend play.
- ** Walks on toes.
- ** Difficulty holding large size crayons.

THIRTY-SIX MONTHS OLD: TYPICAL PLAY

* Feeds self.

* Walks up steps.

* Says at least 3-word sentences.

* Responds to feelings of others.

* Completes 3-4 pieces puzzle.

* Takes turn during play.

* Shows interest in potty training.

Indicators for concern at 36 months:
- ** Words & Speech not understood by others
- ** No interest in other children.
- ** Poor balance, falls frequently.

Those are your indicators for concerns in identifying a special needy child from six months to thirty-six months of age. The first three years of life are so important. That is a description of a baby showing you that later on in life the growth will be just fine. These indicators are a prediction that your child will meet their growth expectations later on in life. It is up to us to recognize these indicators as a starting point for early intervention if needed.

If your child has been on amoxicillin in the past or at this moment - please examine your baby with these indicators to know if your children have been infected with the Amoxicillin Autism Affect. Start right now and observe your baby's play, and see if it matches up with the chart above. It is incredible how I learned so much after what they did to my baby, every day until this moment. But with despair comes hope, and is important to meet hope head on. Every day my baby is involved with something. Today its speech, tomorrow its occupational therapy, and the day after, fine motor skills, gross motor skills, communication therapy, all this hard work and effort on our part is the one ingredient these children need immediately. I promise you that you will see a change and improvement with your babies. Yes, at this early age is when to start the challenge for your baby. My baby has been going through these therapies ever since he came out of the hospital at 15 months old. Today he is six years old at a two-year delayed level.

He does not do things at his age level, only things like that of a four year old, as in the chart above, because of his developmental delay and Autism Spectrum Disorder. If you look at him, he looks just as normal as your regular six-year-old child because of all the hard work that we have applied ourselves to for our baby. So far, it has been a great challenge for us, and it feels like 10 years have passed. In addition, is so important to not let anything stand in your way of achieving a productive goal for your baby, whatever it takes.

As I said before, I cannot stress enough the importance of having your baby evaluated and tested a few times between the ages of 6 months to 36 months old, especially if the baby has been on Amoxicillin antibiotics for all ailments. Ear infections or throat infections, whatever it is, you must have your child tested and compare it with the chart above. In addition, for all the parents who have children between the ages of 4 and 7 years old, who notice that something is not right with their child, it is never too late to have your child tested. I have seen it a thousand times, parents with their inner pride saying "there is nothing wrong with my child." Stop that nonsense! You are doing a great injustice to your child by not having him tested. Perhaps a teacher saw something, or it could be your friend that may see something you cannot. Knowing of all the cycles of Amoxicillin that your child has been taking since birth for his ailments is what is important.

You may be confusing your child's behavior pattern with a normal behavior for a child, as many teachers in our schools think of these children today. But that is another story and another book. I truly suggest that you stop listening to people if they feel otherwise. I say, go right now and get a testing done on your child to see if his growth and development levels are correct. Just do it! You are your child's only hope left for trying to have a productive future for survival if you truly feel something is wrong.

One thing that gets to me is when a teacher notices a child's behavior and they quickly start to label the child as having a behavioral problem, and picking up that behavior from the parents is what they assume to be true, without knowing the facts. That just kills me inside. I hope some teachers are reading this book so they can learn about these children, and they can realize a few things. These children do not have a behavioral problem.

They are special needy children who need teachers to understand them. They are reaching out asking for help. Some are born with disorders, some inherit the disorders through genetics, some catch the disorders from disruption of their immune system by antibiotics, and for the overwhelming population of Autism Spectrum Disorders many develop it from excessive Amoxicillin treatments.

Please have your child tested, because if your child is one among many with this problem, you can seek the proper help for your child and there is plenty of help out there because the system here in America was designed that way. They know how to clean up the mess that they created. Go for it!

11
MY AUTISM BABY

When we first got Christopher to rear him, he was a bundle of joy, and still is. He was two months old at the time. Boy, did we spoil him and still do. Every month we would celebrate his birthday with a cake and a few candles. His face would just light up with a big smile when he saw the candles in the cake. He loved playing patty cake and peek-a-boo, and so did we. He would respond to our every movement.

We would be making different facial expressions, and his response would be with a beautiful smile with those big beautiful eyes, and the longest lashes you can set your eyes on. Those four months before he fell into an ear infection were the happiest time for him and us. His grandma would go crazy over his long eyelashes, and say she wished she had long eye lashes like that. It's funny, but in life we have to be careful when things are so perfect. Then all of a sudden something or someone interferes with your baby's immune system and his anatomy.

Now life gets a little ugly; like what they did to my baby. Today he is Developmental Delayed and Autistic. Survival takes over and the baby's entire future has been altered into a difficult type of view in his mind, as my Baby Boo is suffering today.

<u>His inner self Identity</u> has been changed, which will affect his communication skills.

His Emotional Development including stress, anger, and joy will be confused inside his brain.

His Social Play will be affected including interaction with other children, as we can see is happening to our Christopher today. Teachers and his peers will misunderstand his Pro-Social Behavior, as Christopher is experiencing today in school.

His Large Motor Skills will be weakening with fear that he may fall or hurt himself, as my baby is suffering today.

His Small Motor Skills have also been affected, though we have seen some improvement based on our hard work with him.

His Cognitive Development has been at a slow progress. His Spoken Language has been a challenge since he did not speak one word until he was four years old.

His Writing and Reading has been a great challenge for us. We work on his reading around the clock. As for his writing, it seems tougher than we thought because he cannot hold the pencil correctly, because of the twisting of his fingers.

His Imagination by far has been the most productive so far in our teachings with him.

His Art Skills are just scribble and scrabble because he cannot grasp the crayon correctly, and his neurotransmitters are not like yours and mine. My Autistic baby is suffering these things today. His communication skills and all other skills have been interfered with forever, and are so important to try to reclaim some of these skills. Is up to me to try to readjust him to a completely new outlook for him and his future. We saw a big change in him after he came out of the hospital. No eye contact, always zoning out and staring at something that was not there. Meltdowns occurred about just about anything that was not pleasant to him especially in comprehension. He would go into a meltdown because he just did not understand, and he could not speak to tell me.

This, of course, was very sad to us. We had to teach ourselves the tools and the foundation of working with our baby on his level. He could not speak a word or show any interest on anything, not even baby programs, not even interest in JoJo and Dora which was his favorite program. We knew that we had to work quickly and prepare a foundation for his learning abilities with a short time of early intervention left. It is important to try to catch and identify the spectrum disorders that he may have as young as possible. Those nine months on amoxicillin had changed his whole life.

Today with hard work my wife and I have and will continue to help our baby improve as much as possible, letting him know that he is not alone in his struggles and that Papa and Momma will always be there for him. Children with Autism, young or old, their world is a bit confusing and they are insecure so they quickly and constantly always want to hear those words, "I love you". They always want to be next to you; they do not believe in creating space like you and me when we were their age. Space to these children is frightening. If they do not see you, they cry aloud your name and say, "Where are you Ma-ma Poppa," until the point of seeing you again. These children with ASD cannot survive fear by themselves. The child with the right skills who is not ASD will conquer fear head on, because that is what he learns and sees everyday through the challenges that lie ahead for him in society, but not with Autism Children.

The child with ASD cannot come to that comprehension to meet the child's challenges that are available for every child his age, so this is just one form of his inability to perform an important task that all children his age normally go through in a child's life. This is why it's so important to catch the description of children's disorders whether it be ASD, DD, ADHD as young as possible, and as soon as possible, so you can help them with the proper education and skills that will help their productiveness in society as they grow older.

This is a completely new career for you—a completely new way of life for the parents. A completely new way of thinking from the way you were or what you wanted out of life, and you must be ready to accept the new change in your life, because we love our children. We love them, we reared them and we will always be with them, especially when they feel that we are the only security blanket they have. Ask God for strength - He will give it to you. When my baby was two yrs. old, we started to communicate with him through sign language because he did not speak. Sure enough, he communicated with that because that was something out of the norm for him. By the time he was three years old he managed to understand the - "I love you" hand signs, and of course the "wanting more" hand signs. Communicating was hard for him because he did not speak and it made him mad, so he would react in anger. It would just kill me seeing the sadness on his face telling me how much he wanted to talk. Then a miracle breakthrough came on the week of his birthday at school.

At 4 ½ years old, he just broke out repeating everything that he was listening to all around him. Our hearts just filled with joy hearing him talk back in school. I remember that special word after plenty of speech therapy - "Pa-pa", at the age of 4 ½; it was a wonderful day for us. How I waited to hear those words. Today at almost six years old, he speaks a mile a minute with complications, but still he forces himself because he wants to be like other boys his age.

Of course, he does not connect with sign language anymore, but still I am grateful for that sign language because that was the beginning of opening up his mind to communication. Therefore, it took 54 months to hear him say "Pa-pa". My heart flew to the skies with tears. His speech and words are slurred, but one can come to understand him, which was a good thing. He hesitates every few words, and takes it very slow before finishing each word so he can hear his sounds clearly.

He does not like to be interrupted, even though he interrupts all the time. I was happy to see that the sign language finally came to a halt. He is a bright young boy with his whole life in front of him, and is not worrying about anything because grandma and grandpa will always be there. However, I worry about his future and what I can give him. I have the power of prayer and I am sure the Lord will help me as time goes by. He still lines up his little toys in a straight line. He still bumps his head into things.

His comprehension of things or having patience is below grade level. He is a little over two years delayed and high functioning because of all the work we have provided. I have a problem with the people in society when they look at his meltdowns, which at home or in public people would look and say "that he doesn't look developmentally delayed or that he has autism spectrum disorder—that it's just a behavior problem". They say that my problem may be that the boy lacks discipline and may have a behavior problem; and of course, they would look at me as if I am a lousy parent!

How dare these people, and how lucky they are, of course, because they do not have a special needy child at home. I educated myself of people that do not know about these types of Autistic Children. We as a family must learn how to communicate in teaching society about special needy children. Of course, we cannot blame some people in society because they are innocent for not understanding the truth about these children. They should take the time to learn about what Autism is, and I hope they pick up this book so they can see. Like many people and myself, if I were knowledgeable about Amoxicillin before my baby landed in the hospital I would have never given my baby Amoxicillin.

If indeed I would have picked up a book relating to this story, to learn about the unnoticed Amoxicillin Autism Affect, which caused his immune system and other vital organs to alter, I'm sure I would not have allowed these pediatricians to prescribe Amoxicillin to my baby.

My friends tell me not to blame myself; after all I was under orders by his pediatricians so therefore I'm innocent because I didn't know any better. But that is hard for me, as I am eaten up my guilt every day. Today my baby looks like a fine young man, who does not comprehend certain things you tell him, unless you show love and comfort at the same time. With autistic children, showing understanding and love is all they have to see, to react to your request of calming down from a meltdown, or when it's clean-up time.

Communication comes in all forms of character from within us that we create in order to communicate with our children's level of imagination, to create a communication dialogue. We teach him manners, and he learned how to pray, and he recites it every time we have dinner. His favorite program was called - Developmental Programs for Babies on the Baby Net-Work satellite station. Of course, this program is for younger children. Today he has meltdowns, but we manage to handle his meltdowns with a great big hug and caress him with security, and it works most of the time. What you don't want to do is grab him by the hand and yell at him or her to stop the meltdowns or you'll take away his goodies if he does not want to try and calm down his meltdowns. These exercises of restraint must be abolished from your plan in helping your child, or rather in calming you down as a parent with a special needy child. The way to get through to these children is to come down to their level with love and compassion. Later, when the smoke clears, you can talk with him about the meltdowns; see what excuses he gives you.

It's a great way of communication coming down to these children's level. My grandbaby leaves me speechless with his excuses, but not all his words are connected right so his grammar is a little slow, but I can see he is so bright and smart. His speech and social interaction may not be all there, and he may have meltdowns, but the interest for intelligence is there buried inside of him. He has a photographic-like memory or maybe he just remembers what is important to him, but the fact is that he has a sharp memory.

He does not use a pencil or crayon correctly because of sensory or tactile ability in his fingers is a little unbalanced. He is lovable and friendly, which is something I have to be very close to because in our society today you have sicker brains out there that hurt and kill children. These should be shot Mafia-Style! I personally believe that the laws in this country are too soft in protecting the culprit who victimizes children even until death.

They should give those crazy minds the death penalty without question for crossing the line on a child's life, but that is fantasy. This is the battle and challenge we have as parents. Keeping them safe will be a daunting task, making sure that you know where they are every second of the day and for years to come, but that is O.K. because it will be a wonderful task to complete. We will make it comfortable along the way in order to complete this obligation. We make the best for ourselves and loved ones in order to function with these new readjustments. We must be able to give our autistic children the special understanding that goes the extra mile that they need.

A good reminder is to remember that there is a new sheriff in town in our homes - which is your Baby-Boo or Baby Dee, who needs your love and understanding beyond the norm. My little Boo-Boo smiles a lot and always wants Pa-Pa's attention. He does everything in a routine, something that may annoy you, but you must understand it is his way of life which you cannot change but must help him to adjust. As parents working with your special needs child, you cannot forcibly change his routine thinking that taking away his routine may help him later in life; that is a big No, No.

I have read many stories to that affect and later the parent regrets it. If you change his routine, he will fall into the confusion of mixed calculations. While he is doing things in routine that he is comfortable with, his mind is working at a million things—starting with calculations of everything around him. Having routines for himself helps him understand things better than you think. In addition, do not forget that by changing his routine he will fall into a deep meltdown because he feels that you are interfering with his progress and violating his special space. Every time my baby lines all the toys in a straight line, he gets excited and jumps for joy running and grabbing my hand and saying, "look at what I did, dad. My heart would just fill with joy, and I tell him what a great job he did! The look on his face says it all with a big beautiful smile. This is why you cannot change his routines; his mind is on a mission of learning through the only thing he has left: his imagination. Please make a note of that! These children are in constant contact within their brain function.

Always wanting something, whether the interest or intent is for touching or keeping, or looking or jumping. It will get better as they get older, trust me on this. They begin to see things later than usual, no matter how long or when, they will get there, and that is what we want. They want to be wanted. Books are a big plus, because they love looking at books which will grow into a bigger interest once they see their favorite characters on books, and he's going to want them all which is a good thing.

When Christopher was 4 ½ years old, he liked playing patty-cake and peek-a-boo at that age, something that he missed in his earlier years when he was 2 years old. Does it upset me? No, we love playing it too. We know Boo-Boo will never be 100%, and we know that the older he gets he will show other red flags of a survival function, and we will be there to show him where he went wrong and how to do things. We must never turn our backs on these children, be it as it may. Whatever circumstances are at hand that may bother you, you must fix it ASAP, you must repair it so you can continue the challenge that God left in your hands. The work can be unbearable and relationships between spouses will fall, but these are the qualifications that we need to help them survive. Spouses must see each other to look into your hearts from the moment they fell in love with each other, and start the understanding from that point to be able to work with one another for a child's future that has ASD.

I have read many stories on parents doing the Splits-Ville, and you people just have to stop that. These children need mom and dad together. Right now God wants you people to join hands with love and take care of your baby who has a special need. God understands things are rough, but all he wants is for you to use him for services and strength, and the decision is yours. But life goes on, and if some of you break up your marriage over your child's illness, then I strongly suggest that you never turn your backs on your child.

He will need both of you if he or she has any hope of improving for their survival. It's hard I know, and my heart goes out to all of you, especially the grandparents who hardly have any rights to the hard work of rearing your grandchildren. The laws protecting and enacting for the grandparents of the United States should be more than enforced; they should have been in existence all ready! These poor grandparents worked hard all their lives to retire, and now they're rearing their grandchildren, spending their retirement years on their grandchildren. Is it fair? No! Who said life would be fair, that is why we have the strength of God. The lawmakers of this country should stop the nonsense already. This is old news; the public has been asking for rights for the grandparents for years, we should have rights. I guess for now we have to keep faith alive. My faith, it keeps me going with Boo-Boo, things will get better.

Every day he treats me like a tree, he starts by grabbing my pants then my shirt, and then he continues climbing until he reaches the top of my head, then I cannot see because he wraps his hands around my eyes while sitting on my shoulders. By now I should feel a little calm watching him grow and giving him the tools he needs for a more productive tomorrow, but I can't help but feeling bad, especially in regard to his writing abilities.

His fingers need adjustment in the holding process, and he needs to feel the attachment between the pencil and the paper so he can understand that it is another way of expressing himself. We plan to have him tested for "Dysgraphia." Dysgraphia is a learning disability in children. Many children with ADHD, DD, Autism and other developmental disorders suffer this problem, I see it in his eyes that it hurts him not to be able to write, and that is o.k. that he hurts because it's building up his will every time he tries to write, and that is a good thing. Whatever it is, whatever it takes, and whatever change I must do for my baby I will make happen. Sometimes I look at him, and I thank God that he is alive and happy, we could have lost him. Now is the time.

Time to try to seek justice for my little Boo-Boo, and when I am finished I would hope that I managed to save as many children as I can save from having babies being diagnosed with ASD after a good birth. There is so much to learn and understand, and we have to take it a day at a time. With our children and spouses, it's love that will conquer all obstacles that stand in your way to achieve something so great for your child, and it's right in front of you……………………………….**LOVE**.

12
NO JUSTICE FOR CHRIS

It is clear to me that the families of the 1980s whose children fell victims to the Amoxicillin Autism Affect did not file any lawsuits to proclaim the malpractice negligence against the misuse of Amoxicillin that caused their children's autism in this country.

The government failed those families in question and their children's diseases caused by excessive Amoxicillin for bureaucratic reasons, with the excuse of insufficient evidence, but just the word of the parent. However, the fact is that most of the families from that time could not afford an attorney. It is not uncommon today, because it's true, one would need a dream team to take this force down that has been harming our children for over 30 years. When my grandbaby was six months old he had an ear infection.

When he was 15 months old he landed in the hospital almost dead with 9 months of Amoxicillin in his system. When he was 18 months old Dec. 2005, he was classified Developmentally Delayed. When he was a little over 2 years old Sept. 2006 he was diagnosed with Autism Spectrum Disorder. Shortly after, it was time to take legal action against these pediatricians for what they created that almost took my baby's life. It was time to send them a message. I live in a small town, population about 150,000. Because of conflict of interest, I need to get an attorney outside this little town where everybody knows everybody. When you live a small town, your concerns and complaints should always go out of town, far from town.

Therefore, that is what I did. First stop – "For the People, Morgan and Morgan Law." After making the phone call and speaking with a paralegal about this unbelievable malpractice case, I could not believe the unbelievable story that I got in return.

After explaining to her my case, she told me that they cannot do anything for me unless I have a lot of money to pursue the case, which I did not have. The paralegal attorney whom I spoke with explained to me the new laws on malpractice when suing any doctor especially in Florida. She rather broke everything down briefly.

After talking with her, I did my research. I found myself very upset and disgusted to realize that every time I saw our ex-president speak over the air, on the news, you would always here the remark lawsuits, and now his new laws has touched my family's life in a most criminal way.. The lawmakers signed over a bill making it difficult and much harder to sue doctors in this country over malpractice cases. This was very depressing to hear. Now it would be very difficult to win a case pro-bono unless the victim dies. The other factor would be to prove if the malpractice would cause permanent damage in the future. Without proving that information, even if you know that the doctors are the cause that your baby landed in the hospital almost dead, which reflects a great amount of gross negligence, you can't sue on negligence alone unless the victims dies. Now you need to prove that the negligence will cause permanent damage forever even though he almost died in the hospital. Moreover, what kind of damage is it?

In addition, if you can get a doctor to confirm the permanent damage, which in some cases would be very hard to prove because the future is not here yet. The last factor would be that the law has put the amount of money to be awarded with a dollar amount cap on malpractice cases as in my case. The amount allowed will not provide enough to pay the attorney's bill. However, if you are rich with my problem of doctors putting your baby in the hospital, it would be easy to get justice and you would not care about collecting damages because winning the case and helping millions of children in the process would be worth more than money.

You see, the majority of the victims of the Amoxicillin Autism Affect in this country are of those less fortunate families that could only seek justice from attorneys who accept pro-bono cases. We in society appreciate that, because besides the few dollars that are awarded to the victims for their survival, their main intent is to seek justice regarding what was done to their child. However, that privilege in finding a pro-bono attorney was taken away from yours truly by your own government. A case like mine where the doctor put my baby almost dead in the hospital was an acceptable negligence case with or without future permanent damages, because it was wrong for these doctors to do such a thing to my baby and my family. For now, I can say that these doctors escaped a visit to the court. It hurts to say that today in America any doctor can put your baby in the hospital almost dead, and gets away with it if you do not have a dream team to pursue the case.

I was told that no lawyer in this country would touch my case because of the new laws against malpractice cases. I could not believe what I heard after all the diagnoses that almost killed our baby. Even All Children's Hospital told us how crazy it was for any doctor or pediatrician to give a baby of 6 months of age Amoxicillin for 9 months over an ear infection. This was an infection that never went away, and even my baby's immune system has been compromised forever. I decided to get a second opinion.

My mind started to go crazy with disbelief. I lost count of the attorneys here in Florida that I contacted. I had exhausted my mind and all my energy to learn that my baby has no chance for justice. Even his civil rights have been violated, with no concern for the healthcare of our children. Every attorney told me the same thing—that my baby has a great case but no one would touch it after Mr. Bush changed the laws. If I would of come to them before the new laws, I would have had a multi-million dollar claim against the pediatricians who did this to my baby. Just to quote another attorney she explained her inability to assist me is in no way a comment on the merits of my case, another attorney may be able to assist me and she urged me to contact other attorneys immediately. She explained that such a case as mine has a Statue of Limitation, that if it runs out I will lose my right to sue. She tells me, being that she does not represent me, she cannot tell me when my statute will expire. How crazy does that sound?

Have to hire her first before she can tell me when my limitation runs out, when all I have to do is look it up in the computer. It seems that everything that is coming my way sounds crazy, but is all true. In reality, you cannot even trust attorneys. What kind of country do we really live in when justice goes against our children's healthcare? Why do they do these things to children, woman, and families? She tells me like every other attorney has told me, to file my complaint with the Florida Agency for Healthcare Administration if I cannot get an attorney for my case.

So here I am lost and confused thinking of these doctors getting away with everything, even almost killing my baby. What do I do? Then if I go out of my mind, and say to myself I am thinking bloody vengeance, then I am the bad person! I will be wrong, and I will be declared the crazy one, not the doctors that are killing children— that almost killed my baby! However, I am not a criminal. This is the lifestyle of disgust that we the idiots of this country have allowed this government to be created through greed, money, and power over the people. So what should I do? O.K.

I can't seek justice for my baby, so let me do the next thing and take the advice from all these attorneys that have turned me down for pro-bono, and start writing letters to the proper agencies so they can take hold of this case, and penalize and punish these doctors where it hurts. My first contact and my first letter to the Department of Health July, 2007. In the complaint, I was so detailed I related the entire story from the moment we met the doctors, until the end when my grandbaby contracted the Amoxicillin Autism Affect.

After they reviewed my complaint, I received a reply a few weeks later. An investigation specialist from the Consumer Service Unit of the Department of Health told me that they will be reviewing my complaint. She stated in her letter that it's the mission of the Department of Health, Division of Medical Quality Assurance to protect the public through healthcare licensure enforcement and information. Her letter sounded promising and I felt a relief to know that I am finally going to get some type of justice for my baby.

Hopefully save millions of children from being mistreated by these doctors with Amoxicillin. Days passed into weeks. Then I received a reply three weeks later from Mrs. T saying that they hired a Medical Consultant to review our complaint, and they have determined from his review that the healthcare practitioners of my complaint has not violated the laws or rules that regulates his/her profession.

"Therefore, no further action can be taken," end quote. This was the final straw, how crazy does that sound coming from our own government's Department of Health. This cannot be happening. I quickly fell into a depression beyond the normal. My doctor had to give me pills to calm me down. My life just shut down, and I was ignoring my family, my grandbaby, and my wife.

My wife had to do everything by herself with no aid from me, because my head was spinning every day. After two weeks of despair, I had to look for more options. Therefore, I decided to fight back and I wrote a letter to the State Surgeon General. I felt that if there was anyone that could set the record straight it would come from the State Surgeons General's office.

I wrote them a complaint about the decision that was made from the Florida Dept. of Health, about the nine months of Amoxicillin that was prescribed for my grandbaby by his doctors, which almost killed him. Soon after, I received a letter from them saying that the Health Department acted according to the regulations. Now I had a new fight on my hands. It was not so much that these doctors almost killed my baby, it was worse than that. It is the Government and the Department of Health who is behind all this corruption against our children; letting doctors infect our children with over excessive Amoxicillin that shows signs of the Autism Affect, because it's the Dept. of Health that told me that these doctors did nothing wrong.

Is the government responsible for allowing doctors over medicate our children with Amoxicillin with excessive treatments? One can say that after I told the government of everything that had taken place with my grandbaby, they told me in more words than one, that over 34 cycles of antibiotic in 9 months was O.K. if the doctor chooses to do so. They said it's not wrong because that it's the doctor and he knows what is best for my children.

After I gave them a complete detailed account of what happened to my baby, being in the hospital with 34 cycles of Amoxicillin in his system in just nine months, even after telling them about the bloody bud cheeks around the rectum, blood in the eyes, everything, and the fact that my baby was diagnosed with Developmental Delay and Autism Spectrum Disorder after this clinic of horror experience, they still said that these doctors did nothing wrong!

Nothing wrong! However, there are doctors and professional agencies mentioned in this book saying how crazy they are to over-medicate our children with Amoxicillin that will cause developmental problems in growth. Of cause, now it was more personal than ever with me. After I received the reply from the Health Dept, my mind went crazy. I just could not believe how they would allow this to happen to children and families of America, this so-called great country of ours. This only spells out one thing - that our own government is protecting Amoxicillin and the pharmaceutical companies and doctors in this country. That day my eyes said it all, and it was time to go and get some kind of revenge toward these doctors who think in their sick minds that they got away with what they did to my baby. My wife looked at me and knew that I was not feeling well. I told her that day that I loved her, and never to worry about any problems because I was going to be next to her for the rest of her life.

She looked at me with a sad face as if she knew I was out for revenge. I quickly left the house, jumped in my car and took off like a bat out of hell. I was driving recklessly throughout the area and was not afraid to get stopped by a cop. Fact is, if a cop would have stopped me back then, I would not be writing this book today. I drove my car and double parked the car in front of the clinic. I left my keys in the ignition and slammed the door open to the clinic. It was a full house but I was not paying attention. I walked right up to the window and asked to speak to Dr. Marlin.

The secretary told me that he was out that day, but I could see another doctor if I like. I asked to see Dr Marlene she's the one that told us that my baby did not need to go to the emergency room a few days before he landed in the hospital almost dead. At that moment I felt someone grabbing onto my pants, I turned and saw a little baby boy, that looked a little baby angle, a beautiful little boy he was. Then suddenly my mind just woke up from this bloody vengeance that entered my mind; at that moment I looked around my surroundings because of this cute little person. The people in the waiting room saw how much I was sweating. Then in a flash, I saw the little boy looking at me, and he looked like if he was very sick, and I just ran out of the clinic, jumped into my car and drove away. As I was driving home, for a moment I just wanted to end my life, because of what I allowed to happen to my baby, and I started crying like a baby, hitting my head and wondering *what am I going to do now for justice for what they did to my baby?*

How can this government allow this to happen to our children? I started thinking what logic God would have me use. Of course, I got rid of the idea of giving the doctor a beating, because in reality I am not a criminal. After the long drive home getting my head together, I managed to calm down with my senses. As I entered my home I just grabbed my grandson in tears, kissed my wife and went on to my office, put the computer on and cried some more.

The next day after I calmed my mind down, I decided to write to our Governor. After all, he was always talking about how much he values children. Writing to an agency is one thing, but writing to the Governor is another matter. I wrote everything in the letter to the Governor for help. I explained detail by detail even about some of the information in this book, and I pleaded for his help. On June 13, 2008, he finally answers my letter after a long wait, with his Office secretary of Citizen Services. She told me in the letter – "Thank you for contacting the governor. The governor appreciates your concern for your grandson's healthcare and safety and the governor has asked me to respond on his behalf." She tells me to assist me better; she forwarded a copy of my letter to the Department of Health, Division of Medical Quality Assurance for review and response.

However, she already knows that I have contacted the Dept. of Health because it is in the letter I mailed to the governor. She then tells me in the letter - "You do have the option to pursue this case by contacting an attorney."

However, she knows I have already done that, and the governor knows about the new malpractice law that passed, or I would not be writing to the governor for help! She then said in the letter, the Constitution limits the governor's intervention in the matters that should be resolved through the court system. What does that mean? What? What does this mean to all families that have gone through what I have? How can something like that be said to any Floridian and to all families. Being that there is a constitution written about the obligations of our governor, it gives me great pleasure to tell you how I feel about it with no prejudice in the making

Let us break Down What the Governor's Secretaries Statement Means to Me and Many Other Floridians: She already knows that the Health Department is wrong, In addition, she knows the legalities behind this case and she does not want our esteemed governor involved with this case involving children. Alternatively, maybe he does not even know about my letter of complaint. On the other hand, maybe he does not really care.

Alternatively, maybe he just said things that people wanted to hear just so he could be elected. Even our governor! With this rejection comes many maybes or rather someone has the wrong interpretation of the Constitution for our governor? Our governor has the right to get involved with any matters pertaining to our babies and children that involves allegations about his Department of Health allowing an antibiotic to harm our children.

This is one of the reasons why we elected him governor! He is our governor for problems like this one involving his administration and the children of Florida. Fact is, the governor is there for the people and by the people, and for his secretary to tell me that the constitution limits the governor's intervention in the matters that should be resolved in court, it's crazy to me! She is right about resolving a problem like mine in court, but I cannot find a lawyer to take the case, so I decided to take the problem to him, after all, he is our children's governor and is supposed to be an advocate to these children.

What kind of governor did we put in office with such a cold heart? Another example of how blind we've become, choosing the wrong candidate for office. Trusting everything he is telling us that he will do for the people turns to be a lie; a perfect replica of trusting your pediatrician with amoxicillin that will not hurt the baby's system, turns out to be worst than a lie. It seems to me that the secretary of the governor's office does not realize the true responsibilities our governor must have for our children. In addition, as far as our court system goes for problems like mine and other victimized children, in recent years lobbyists for the health care industry and the insurance industry have persuaded our legislature to enact laws designed to discourage patients and their attorneys from making claims against health care providers. It seems that every time in the past before the new medical malpractice law came into effect, I always noticed President' Bush's State of the Union address, making some kind of remark talking junk medical malpractice suits of some kind, so I guess that my case was just junk medical malpractice.

The new law has substantially increased the time, efforts and expenses required to investigate and prosecute claims. As I've stated earlier, the doctors gave 34 cycles of antibiotics in 9 months that put my baby in the hospital almost dead. Then, 4 months later he was diagnosed with Autism Spectrum Disorder & Developmentally Delayed. A case like this will cost a great deal of money to investigate and put together as well as limiting in many cases the amount of money that a patient may recover in a civil lawsuit.

Unfortunately, this means that in a large number of cases with perfectly valid claims, attorneys will not touch the case. So you see Miss Secretary of the Governor, the only hope of justice that all these children and their families have is the governor. Please remember that if you're reading this book. After so much news on children catching the ASD & DD disease in this country, it took almost the death of my grandbaby to prove finally to the governor and the Health Department how is this happening to our children. Not one official or our Governor agreed to see the truth of the matter; they completely ignored my claim. I guess I am a nobody to them. Whether they like it or not, I found out why this country has been witnessing the high rise of Autism Spectrum Disorder & Developmental Delay at 1 in 88 children. I found out the truth. What these doctors did was beyond negligence to give a 6-month-old baby for the next 9 months, 34 cycles of Amoxicillin, landing him in the hospital almost dead. The baby's immune system and intestines had been compromised forever causing a change in the baby's development unbelievable.

I also found out that many great doctors and researchers have concluded positive results against the Amoxicillin Autism Affect on our children. All you people that are reading this book, all you have to do is put the dots together. I even get turned down for help by my own government, and almost all State Agencies involving the healthcare of our children here in America. Whom can I talk with? Where can I go for justice, if any?

If I had money, I would hire the dream team attorneys. Not only would I win the case, the dream team would make sure that this does not happen to another child. They will also make sure to stop all Amoxicillin doctors that have hurt children, and have gotten away with it because of the new malpractice act. The laws will eventually change to reform the Malpractice Act, because it cannot last forever having doctors do what they feel like, and at the same time harming our children protecting their interest.

The Malpractice Act must change to benefit the people and not the doctors once again. The numbers of sick and infected infants and children are growing quicker than we imagine, with doctors and pediatricians getting away with prescribing excessive medicines. You the people, families of all lifestyles - you are stronger than you think. Remember together we stand and divided we will continue to see our children growing in number breaking records, developing Developmental Delay with the Amoxicillin Autism Affect.

After my research, I will say it again, I cannot stress it enough to you readers that there is another division of Autism. The Autism that you are born with, we understand its creation, but the Autism that is diagnosed within five years after a good birth, is in question, which includes a high number of children coming from the Amoxicillin Autism Affect population. This is the Autism that is created by doctors through Amoxicillin and other antibiotics, or what ever medicine that has been use randomly throughout on the baby. A time limit to activate a disease that will harm our children forever.

This government has allowed these doctors to administer the drug of choice to infants and children over an ear infection, throat infection and other ailments; and this is causing major problems within the child's system. These Antibiotics kill your good bacteria that our body needs, harming and interfering with the baby's immune system causing different types of infectious bacteria that interferes with brain development resulting Developmental Delay and Autism Spectrum Disorders later on in the child's life. All because the drug of choice for ear infections and throat infections is Amoxicillin; which is the number one drug that is harming our children. For the reasons of profit and gain they will not discontinue using Amoxicillin on babies and children. We are living in a crazy society when we allow these crazy doctors and pediatricians to continue to harm our children in this one area of Autism that they will suffer for the rest of their lives.

We have to understand that taking Amoxicillin for an ear infection on a baby is not the answer. The problem is that most doctors currently enjoy giving the baby excessive antibiotics like Amoxicillin, why? No one really knows why? In addition, it seems that no one really cares. All we can do is guess because our government does not care about our concerns. We can only assume as to why. The more drugs sold, the higher the stock and the more money they earn. However, we all know now that Amoxicillin can harm the baby more than curing the baby from pain.

This is important, that all new parents read this book; parents with new born babies, parents with children. Buy this book as a gift. Don't let them hurt your baby. I have gone through all the right steps for justice and failed my grandbaby. What good am I for my grandbaby? Can you even imagine how I feel at the moment? You the people, families, grandparents, you are part of the reason why I am writing this book, in hopes that my grandbaby's message and our mission will prevail in justice for your children and my little Boo-Boo. Therefore, I will continue my challenge in helping my baby see a better tomorrow. I will do everything in my power to have this book published. It's the only chance for justice I have left is to tell the world what happened to my baby, and the same thing can happen to your baby as it has in the past to many families.

I hope that the message in this book can convince influential people who are reading this book to do something about the health regulations if we do not put a stop to the #1 drug that is administered to our children from every pediatrician in America - "Amoxicillin." It will destroy the future of this country. It may be o.k. for you and me to kill our infections because our system can handle the abuse, but on an infant and children - it can kill them, or hurt them, and turn your baby Developmental Delay and Autism Spectrum Disorder for the future of this country..................It's A Fact!

13
I'M SORRY FOR YOUR LOST

Let's be real, let's be honest, every time we experience a love one, ourselves, or our children, going through a procedure from your doctor at the hospital you have to sign a document. This document states the hospital or doctors whom performed the procedure are not liable for any mishaps resulting in death or any other such events from the procedure being done.

We go ahead and sign the document or they will not conduct the procedure. In some cases, the patient does not make it. The focus of course is the patient system was weak, not enough of this or that; an accident has occurred, death by accident. It is sad to see the #1 drug of choice recommended by every pediatrician in the US, used on ear infections and any other type of aliment on infants and on our children, destroying our babies system.

The medical community is always protected even in wrong doing.

It is clear to see; any pediatrician can take your six-month-old infant baby, and use that baby as a guinea pig to their amoxicillin long term experiments, as they did to my baby! It has changed the way I feel about pediatricians in this country. I have to be very careful with pediatricians head on, when it comes to my baby. They can very easily kill your baby using the hands of parents, and just say to you accidents do happen. Believe me when I say, it does happen. As we have seen many unconcerned professionals are getting away with diverse crimes in our society, and over excessive antibiotic death is no exception. The pediatrician has two things to go on: 1 - They can kill the pain 2 - They can cure the problems with antibiotics; but is that the answer for a proper cure? And if so, it has left evidence that its not, evidence of inner destruction on babies without informing.

If they kill your baby with medication, for them it's just a margin of error that would be corrected by saying - it was an accident, I'm sorry for your lost. They pay you restitution if you can file a lawsuit against them. A margin of error that should not be ever allowed or accepted. When this happens, it seems that a thousand doctors all of a sudden come up with new excuses, new answers as to why it happened?

This doctor says one thing, the other doctor says another thing, while another doctor who wrote a book on bad medicines says that they are all wrong, that he is right. Who is right? Who is wrong? Whom do we listen to? It is crazy! Think about that for a moment: a pediatrician or any other doctor can actually make these mistakes with your child's diagnosis or medicine, and forget that oath, and forget that there is no room for error when it comes to your child's life. Here is something that may affect your child for the rest of their lives, and the doctors will get away with it. When this occurs, the parent will take the blame in the eyes of the medical community and our government as not being aware of your child's condition. History has shown us malpractice cases that entails a pediatrician or medical doctors who has committed the deadliest decisions in their profession by taking a baby's life accidentally or intentionally. The doctor is in the driver's seat and your children are the passengers with no seat belts if the doctor has an accident! It's old and serious news. News that we do not take seriously enough. News that we do not bother to listen or learn by.

What do we learn when we hear about cases like these? Do we parents learn by making wiser decisions when it comes to dealing with pediatricians on our baby's behalf? I do not think so, because we trust our good pediatricians; we say, "Oh, she is a great doctor to my little princess." Alternatively, do we ignore what we see on the news about Dr. Death who has taken another mother's or baby's life? Unfortunately, we ignore these stories, and continue living our lives without having any fear of our own pediatricians who take care of our baby's healthcare.

Peaches and cream thinking dictates that it will never happen to your baby because he or she is a good pediatrician to your baby. Therefore, we continue to live our lives with no fear. You put most of your energy on hopes and dreams of someday hitting your mark of success; then comes one day when your time limit is up, when a tragedy does occur with your baby involving the very same pediatrician for whom you have never feared; just like what happened to me.

All because of the trust you have in your pediatricians over your baby's healthcare. Look, I am not saying not to trust your pediatrician; what I am saying is not to put all your trust on your pediatricians over your baby's healthcare, and to have more awareness and alertness to your pediatricians' performance when they recommend Amoxicillin for your baby, or any other antibiotic that can harm your children's system.

If indeed you become aware of your baby's developmental changes after a few years, a red flag should pop up in your head, that is the time to get serious and look for some answers after this tragedy occurs in your baby's life. Now that the situation is changed, what do you do now? You walk among the many families that have lost their children through death from Amoxicillin, or have been harmed through the very doctors who have been prescribing this drug to your baby—this doctor that's supposed to care so much for your child.

Now you can join the sideline of pain, confusion, and misery, because that is all you can do for now besides suffering your regrets. So now you go through life kicking yourself saying - "I should have been more vigilant with myself about our baby's pediatrician's decision making when it came to our baby's safety." Then of course, the tragedy and loss will haunt you for the rest of your life, walking in pain and sadness. Of course, I do not hope or wish this destruction on you and your child, and may God bless you and your families.

It's sad to say that there are many families including myself on the sideline walking in pain and despair. I'm sorry, but this is how it is. All that I have mentioned to you so far is the truth, and it's important that you do not forget what you are reading in this book even if you do not agree - look it up yourselves. How many babies suffer and have passed away in death, leaving mommy and daddy behind?

If you start doing an in-depth research of Amoxicillin accidents and children, you will find there is not enough room in your memory banks, or enough paper to come up with an answer of cases. There are too many to keep records of. That is how serious the problem is. I could remember a time when you or your family was sick, doctors used to do house calls. They came with their little black bag to your doorstep. The bill was always moderate to fit your needs or the doctor would say forget about it, putting compassion into his work.

Today compassion, in my opinion, does not exist when it comes to feeding your child as much Amoxicillin they can to fit their bill. I am sorry, but that is the way it is. There was a time when doctors truly cared about helping the people and securing a healthy community around them. For the community family doctor it was never about money—only his community and your family's healthcare. Back then, if you were a medical doctor, you were respected and honored by the work you did in your community even if you couldn't afford a doctor or antibiotics for the caring heart doctors had for children. The community would look at that doctor as a very special caring person; a gift from heaven. He would be placed on the prayer list in almost every church in town to continue and bless the work he was doing. God Bless the Doctor! Words that would continue around America throughout history until the 1970s. However, today it's a different story. The 1970s marked the start of a new era for the next 39 years in the medical community.

In addition, new research for the ever-growing number of victims of Autism, Cancer, Diabetes, etc. New medical discoveries, new ideas for medical equipment and tools, expansions of hospitals. New policies for Medicaid Medical Health Insurance that were created in 1964. Populations are growing everywhere in this country, more and more people are becoming doctors and nurses for the better of our communities.

There are more schools for our children, more colleges for our medical professionals, new inventions, new antibiotics. The late 1980s marked the beginning of what was to become a multitudinous population of children with Developmentally Delayed and Autism Spectrum Disorder, and the start of the Autism population dilemma that we are witnessing today. The 1980s would show families throughout America challenging doctors on excessive antibiotic such as Amoxicillin since the introduction of the drug during that time. Doctors quickly joined forces all over America claiming that the Autism was genetically based, environmental, and street drugs was another way to have developed ASD is their claim The 80s was also a time when Aids was very common, climbing in the numbers because of the amount of drugs in our streets. In the 1990s parents against vaccines believed that their children may have caught the Autism Spectrum Disorder from the vaccines they gave to their children, not realizing the affects of the antibiotic Amoxicillin they were giving their children. I believe it was a great weapon and excuses were given by the medical community in convincing parents complaining about the Amoxicillin Autism Affect.

The medical community began using the Aids patients as a convincing excuse tactic in the battle of understanding how a normal birth child can contract autism and where it came from. A new excuse was offered, telling those parents with Aids the reason for your child's development - "It's obvious," they said. It was the drugs and Aids. Nevertheless, there is no evidence to support that, only assumptions.

Today is a different matter than past history and the early 1900s. People of all calibers are demanding answers because of the rapid growth population of autism in every class of people. In 2006, 1 in 166, a year later to 1 in 150 children, to 1 in 130, children that were being diagnosed with Autism, as we saw 1 in 110 in 2011, now today 2012 1 in 88. Within the past 4 years alone, the numbers of children with Autism have sky rocketed tremendously.

That number 1 in 88 is a scary number. The production keeps growing without the true explanation of the autism affect we see on children who are born normal, then later with the ultimate diagnose. Now some parents refuse to hear the excuses that the medical community has to offer. The future of our children and our country may be in trouble and affected forever. Until this day, most doctors and most pediatricians still manage to keep that agreement by saying that is hard to say that Amoxicillin is another leading cause of Autism.

After they read this story, is my prayer that God sends an angle to smack their cheeks with some common logic to take out Amoxicillin & Augmentin from every clinic in America; either bring back what was there before or go back to table and create something that will not hurt our children. As for me, and the families of the 80s, we say that the Medical Community and the Government Department of Health have been lying for 30 years about Amoxicillin and children, and now the truth is out of the bag.

Today doctors still say that they need more proof. In addition, the parents are eating it up not realizing that at the same time these doctors giving them all kinds of positive thinking, their babies immune system and digestive tract are being infected with a bacterium build up that will affect their development as time passes. The recipe for the Amoxicillin Autism Affect is on the move of due time. These cycles reach a danger lever that is never explained to the parents. All you have to do is add up in your minds the hundred of thousands of parents that are not informed about this danger level destruction that causes developmental problems, better yet, the millions of parents that are not informed and just see what I see; you want to know where the growing population of autism of 1 in 88 is coming from? The key word to remember here is cycles. We know one thing; a study was done on what some doctors have to say about cycles of antibiotic and the dangers it will bring to our children.

Over twenty cycles of this junk into your baby, you have crossed the lifeline, after twenty two cycles you have crossed the finish line. In my opinion, the reason why many doctors in this country allows this to happen to our children, frankly we will never know for sure. However, one thing is certain: we will be more aware on this subject of the Amoxicillin Autism Affect from here on because you are learning now the way is created. I can only guess at reasons why pediatricians would go so far if indeed they know of these studies with amoxicillin.

Their reasons can be endless, however, I know there are many good caring pediatricians in the medical community with the knowledge of antibiotics and the immune system, and the harm it can cause a baby's system. I also know that the majority of pediatricians do not take the time to look at their patient's history of antibiotics to share with the parents; I got that information from head on experience from my baby's Clinic of Horror Pediatricians Anonymous.

In my opinion, I believe some doctors themselves do not realize that they creating the Amoxicillin Autism Affect upon children. They are hurting our children, eating up the parent's finances, insurance, and they are doing a great job at it. Somebody has to say it!

We have caring doctors that have done research on the subject of Amoxicillin and Autism. They are starting to come out slowly with the truth, because they themselves have a fight on their hands against the multitude of doctors in this country that refuse to be truthful on this subject.

In my opinion some Amoxicillin doctors that do this to children will do anything to stop the truth from coming out, but they're running out of excuses about the issue of Amoxicillin and Autism. Please note that I do not have anything against doctors or pediatricians. I am only against hurting our children for life, with developmental delay and autism through their antibiotic Amoxicillin.

Another past history argument, was Augmentin composed of Amoxicillin that infected our children with autism spectrum disorder and developmental delay in the 1980s and 1990 is claimed by parents in this country from different states. Did we learn our lesson then, no! Who is right, and who is wrong? We have to treat these doctors like a business, as they treat us—with no more trust. No More Trust! Today's medical doctors will not treat you if you are sick unless you have insurance or money to pay for the services, and you can't blame them because they pay bills too, but give me a break! Not all doctors are the same; you just have to be careful, that is all. We have been carrying this trust for doctors since we were children for years. It seems like forever, when all the while we were just a number to doctors. This is how life is today, and it saddens me to know how real this is. Doctors must be kept in our suspicions at all times, and at all cost.

Some of them do not even know the latest research on major diseases, or even new findings for major complications that a patient may have - they just do not know because they themselves have not done their research; they say they don't have the time. Times have changed. It is up to you to do your own research on your illness before you visit any doctor for any problems you may have. When you go to visit the doctor's office for a medical problem that your child may have, be prepared with your research, so you can educate these doctors on your findings.

Even request other options in case you do not approve of the medicine or Amoxicillin that lies ahead for you or your baby. You are in control not your doctor—remember that. Do not let them do the driving anymore, and do not let these doctors become the shotgun driver when it comes to your children's healthcare. One last note to this chapter, I have a question for all you readers - Do you know how many babies and children have died from Augmentine and Amoxicillin since the 1980s, accidental or misdiagnosed until this day?

The stories are sad, and the deaths are one too many. My heart and prayers goes out to those families who have lost their babies and children to this poison. After you see, only then can you put the puzzle and pieces together. You will be convinced regarding the deliberate actions that have been formed against our children in the name of money and profit from the Amoxicillin Autism Affect. Come now; let's review how four doctors from the clinic of horrors, came to the doorsteps of my grandbaby's life, but failed in ending his life.

A Quick Review……………..

December, 2004, the baby is 6 months old. This month of Dec.2004 would be the start of a nightmare for us and for our baby that would last until this day and forever. That month we put our baby's healthcare in the hands of four pediatricians, and a nightmare that would continue to last until the baby landed in a pool of blood in the All Children's Hospital 9 ½ months later. Why it happened is the big question?

The fact is that any story that brings harm to a baby is touching and heartbreaking and Lord knows that there are many. This is the story about my grandbaby that at the time was only a 6-month-old and in good health, and over an ear infection he suffered a very bad journey—a journey of grossnegligence that would lead his life to disaster, and through the black hole of death. But he made it back by the miracle of our Lord God.

I was shutting down my grandson's God-given life, because I was under orders by the doctors to administer a lengthy course of Amoxicillin antibiotic that turned to a crazy experiment of the doctor. Me being grandpa of the year, I was not as knowledgeable as I am today about Amoxicillin. I put all my trust in four pediatricians and their knowledge of quality healthcare when it came to my baby. Until this day, I hate myself and torture my mind in tears after constant remembrance of all the horrible moments my grandbaby spent with me while I had to administer the amoxicillin to him, especially one moment that almost turned deadly for my grandbaby during a horrible time, administering the Amoxicillin in which he almost choked in the process.

This is something that will never leave my mind. I did not know any better at the time but to put my full trust in these doctors, thinking that my baby was going to get the best healthcare for an ear infection. I was wrong in not being intelligent enough for my baby's illness. I will never forgive myself for that! At the same time, I did not know anything about Amoxicillin, antibiotics, or Autism, and Autism Spectrum Disorder for that matter. Honestly, I was stupid to say the least for not being as educated as I am today.

It took this destruction in my baby's life to wake me up. Now, I will finish this book of facts so people themselves can see the truth of 1 in 88. What they did with my baby with Amoxicillin is nothing more devastating then dying from the drug, and my heart goes out to these families who have lost babies and children in the process of this type of treatment. They did to my baby what they did back in the 1980s, when Amoxicillin came crashing in to all pediatricians. After that event, came a time when families from the rising of developmental delay and autism children gave Amoxicillin a failing grade, for being the course of their children's autism. The government stood their ground by saying that the doctors "did nothing wrong." I suggest that all parents start taking notes from now on when visiting your baby's pediatrician. Bring with you a note book and pen. By writing things and events down on paper, even make quotations of who said what, it may someday help you understand certain things.

It will make you see your baby's performance in a timeline, as well as your pediatrician's performance, which in my baby's case with his four pediatricians was a living hell. It is important to realize, that every hospital, every doctor, is protected from any mishaps that we understand to be otherwise. We must follow our hearts and minds for logical answers, and not give in to those who profit and benefit from our mistakes. These are our children, and we will not harm our children's development system any longer with Amoxicillin and its relatives. I am yelling out "stand clear pharmaceutical" – "I'm Sorry for you're lost!"

14
WHERE DOES AUTISM COME FROM

It hurts so much when you cannot come to your grandbaby's rescue, even when he is right in front of you and needs you the most. They say that Autism comes from the genes of the family tree, to environmental factors in our communities and our personal lives. For the genetic part of it, it draws a big question mark, except for the identical twins factor, and of course it is just not possible for the gene unless we are speaking about hundreds of years for one gene to change.

For the natural Autistic child at birth, it is well known that the birth of a child with distinctive attributes that shows development changes has puzzled doctors and researchers since the early 1900s when the medical community first discovered Autism, but in reality, autism has been in existence for hundreds of years, maybe thousands.

However, for the children who are autism who were born normal, then in later years became autism, this group should have never contracted the Autism Affect. We must go into the past, in order to understand the production line of autism throughout the years, and then chronologically find out the source for the mass production we are witnessing today; which is what I have done exactly to get the answers I was looking for. In the early 1900s Autism was first recognized, and the disease started to become of bigger interest to the communities because the disease was hitting well defined families of stature only. Again, autism was recognized more with families of stature than the children of immigrants who were building this country, cold hard laborers and their families. Families of wealth, sons and daughters of prominent families, were the first to contract Autism in great numbers. Imagine that, only children of the rich class, and not the poor. These rich families were also the first to reject the genetic affect idea because they could not pinpoint a family history with the disease.

This, of course, may be a big surprise to many, probably the first time you heard about this Autism news. As for the environmental factors, these rich families in the early 1900s believed that there was more to the story on how their children caught the disease but they could not find any answers, only assumptions. Although in that time, the poor population may or may not have had cases of Autism, it was well known throughout the land that Autism was among the rich families, 'families of stature' they called them.

These rich families were in a world of their own, because they felt far more important than the poor minority families with children without the disease. The differences back then in history to today's autistic children of 2012, our children of this present time are not a majority of prominent rich families of stature, as they were classified in the early 1900s. At this moment in time with a great majority of autism rising high, they come from all lifestyles, rich or poor, with the majority being that of less prominent families and not the wealthy as they described in early history. After my research, I find back then in time, the wealthy families were the only ones that could have afforded a doctor and the modern medicine antibiotics for their families. Modern medicine back then was not an easy handout, with experiments of medicine in all parts. As they experimented with medicine that could cure the children, the community praised doctors, and doctors were hard to come by that dealt with what we call today autism development.

They did not call it autism, but they knew the term "development". A new discovery with no proper research or advance technology to understand a cure or treatment for the abnormal development children, Whether they had a visual defect appearance or they're behavior was that of an un-normal child as they described back then, it was odd to see children of well defined people of stature with this dilemma. They would call them crazies, and lock them up in a room or in a hospital.

They were completely rejected from society. I believe their prize medicines were reserved for people of influence, the wealthy, and doctors had limits on getting these new modern medicines such as antibiotics out to the fortunate ones with money. As for the medicines, if you did not have money to pay for the miracle drug, you had to turn to home remedies, like garlic, natural herbs and oils. However, their home remedies of plants, garlic, herbs would bypass and continue through time into today, as the natural medicine that works for all times. In my opinion their rich man's medicine they gave their children for fevers, runny nose, ear infections would turn out to be the cause for their children's developmental problems. After seeing today's positive studies on antibiotic amoxicillin and developmental delay, one can conclude the cause of early history autism with those children could have been the meds.

Their improper diagnosis would show the children as mentally retarded or schizophrenic having using medicine (antibiotic) involvement for the child's dysfunctional behavior in that time in history, they could not put it together, they could not see the antibiotics was the cause for their autism. You cannot argue with facts. Compare the past thirty years, and the proof being introduce to you right here, antibiotic amoxicillin is the cause of the Amoxicillin Autism Affect today through a deadly cycle transition with antibiotics, like what happen to my baby,.

My baby is suffering today because of it. Now imagine the early 1900s and their medicine with children of stature. Something to think about! Developmental disorders that could never have been properly diagnosed in that time. They did not have the advance knowledge on medicine and the human body as we do today. Today in 2012, for many people including myself it is the Amoxicillin antibiotic and related medicines in the same family to Amoxicillin that are harming our children. Pediatricians are feeding our children, excessive amounts in their systems that are altering our children's developmental state of mind for 30 years - just like in the early 1900s when their antibiotic type medicines harmed the children of people of stature. Is it any wonder why you rarely heard of the poor population being infected with this disease back then? Autism was not classified with the name back then, but instead they thought their children were turning crazy, and eventually they would be placed in an asylum for their protection. Parents did not know how to care for their own child who had Autism.

Their children were being seen as having mental problems years after a good birth, aside from the ones born with a birth defect as we remember the Elephant Man in the nineteenth century. Some assumed that these children's mental problems were caused by lack of parenthood. They blamed parents and treated them as such. A parent used to be fingered out as bad parents in those times, and today is not different. Some people felt that is was the medicines being administered to the child that was causing the problem; of course that would be ruled out by their medical scholars (also by their investors I am sure).

Today the medical community refuses to look into the amoxicillin as a problem to autism, just like in history. After the discovery of these children with developmental problems, this disease later became known as Autism, and the name was finally given. One of the differences from past history's autism children from today's autistic children is that in the early 1900s the number of cases of autism children was so rare that they could not even put a number on how many cases there were. However, the very few they recognized was very disturbing to the medical community in later years. In the 1960s, a quick study was done and it was found that 1 in 2,500 children were being diagnosed with autism, and the medical community was going nuts trying to find an answer as to why. That study in later years would be revised into 1 in 10,000 children, making this disease rare in the making. Today it's growing faster than is imagined, and we must do something about it, to help new mothers to be informed that their children can also contract the same fate.

Something is happening here! Now you have to wonder about the growth of the autism children between the early 1900s and 1960 when they did the study—it was growing slowly. In 1980, only 1 in 10.000 children were diagnosed. Now look at the increase, in 2009, 1 in 110 children being diagnosed. The number of our children has grown into thousands because of the same fate the children of stature in the early 1900s suffered with their antibiotics.

Our children will continue to suffer the amoxicillin autism affect for life, unless the Dept. of Health in our Government orders the pharmaceutical companies to master mind something else for our children other than Amoxicillin antibiotics, and do a complete study on this killing medicine. The medicines given to those children in time was not as over excessive, as the future children that are given over excessive antibiotics in greater numbers and longer cycles; making our modern antibiotics more dangerous and deadly for our children. It is the amount of cycles of feeding that junk that changes the child's development with no recovery. The numbers were very high to the community of the 1960s, with autism on the rise. People started to get alarmed and scared for the children. Even in the 1960s, modern medicine was expensive. A great many families still used home remedies for the cure of an ear infection and other sicknesses.

In 1970s, there was another study done, but more in-depth and found to be 1 in 10,000. For ten years, between 1970s and 1980, that number 1 in 10.000 children with autism stood fast, still making this Autism disorder rare in the making. After passing the Medicaid bill in 1965, medicines was available for every child in the US. As for antibiotics, there were more pharmaceutical companies making the medicine faster than drinking a cup of water.

Apart from all the reasoning that is declared, for me it's fair to say with the information I gathered, between the early 1900s and 1980s, the reason for so many autism child after a normal birth, logically speaking, by feeding the baby antibiotics from infancy to toddler's medicine affecting the child's inner system, from the immune system to the brain. Of course, one cannot deny the group of children who are born autism at birth, one might say just a hand full compare to the greater numbers after a normal birth. Think about it, when the baby gets sick, doctors prescribe medicine to see if the sickness of the child will subside, to see if their experiment with the antibiotic for a cure might just work, like in my case. Every time that same child gets sick, again the same medicine goes into his system; after a period of time with build up bacterium, and then comes a diagnosis of Autism at the age of 3 to 5 years. Over-excessive medication is a prime qualification for doctors to get richer. Pharmaceutical companies always had the approval for limitations when it came to consumption of excessive antibiotics.

Whichever way you want to slice it, I blame pharmaceutical companies for many health tragedies among our babies and children. I am accusing Amoxicillin of being the # 1 medicine of the main causes of an autism affect that is being ignored by our Governmental Dept. of Health and Pharmaceutical Companies for thirty years. They know it! What I would say to you is to join the cause of facts and do your research after reading this book. Join the cause to end Amoxicillin from all pediatrics in America.

If you think that pharmaceutical companies do not know which medicines and that Amoxicillin can cause developmental delay in the mind - think again! We parents have a tendency of being satisfied with the antibiotics that are created. They are so easy to come by and we allow them without concern of compromising our baby's immune system, because we believe in trusting our doctors, and this is a fact!

I am sure that the antibiotics of that time in history were the cause of the autism development in their children, but ignored that avenue like the medical community has done today. For me, that was the birth of - antibiotics & autism - that gradually caused this awful statistic of 1 in 88 children we see today being diagnosed with Autism. Too much junk in our baby's system everyday, year after year. I blame our Government and the Medical Community of the 1980s for not listening to parents about Amoxicillin causing autism on their children. When we go to the pediatrician for our children's illnesses and they prescribe Amoxicillin, we expect the doctor giving this medicine to our children, is treating our children wisely and with the intent to bear no harm to the child.

They were wrong about that! They told us - "If you use the antibiotic the right way it will not hurt the child. Instead, I see how it has injured our children permanently until this day with our children's system being infected and their minds developmental delay. The first 5 years of a child's life is very important to the parent. The preschool of the child will depict his forward ahead to kindergarten, and the healthcare of the child will depict his ability to conquer kindergarten, this is every parents wish come true.

However, it is not that way for most parents. For most of us, our children's first five years of childhood have consumed so many cycles of antibiotics plus amoxicillin that it has been interfering with the capability to conquer the road ahead for public school. They carry spoors of infectious bacterium growing inside of them until the time limit is up for the autism affect to take over. Many children die from it.

You do not hear about the deaths Amoxicillin has caused our babies over the years; why should you hear about amoxicillin causing autism, it is a controlled system. We are walking hypnotized when it comes to our children's health because we have blind faith in doctors. In reality, of all that has been done and said, we should only have our faith reserved for God! I am here with chronological facts that are true about my claim. Again, my main focus is the children who are born normal then in later years turns autism. Let us look at some.

Looking at our history with Autism, and seeing possibilities of medicine for the cause of Autism during that time in history, hitting mostly the rich families, families of stature, one cannot ignore but entertain the thought. Look at the studies of amoxicillin and developmental delay, at the inner destruction from just 20 cycles of amoxicillin in the baby's system. Look at what they did to my son—put it all together chronologically, and the truth is in front of you.

Remember; let the record show that from the 1980s until today 30 years later, autism has grown to 1 in 88 - why? I am here to show you truth, and I hope you are seeing what I'm seeing. The sixty thousand dollar question in my mind is "Why? Why is the medical community letting this happening to our children today?" Today, doctors have stood their ground, saying that somehow there must have been someone in the family genes with autism and developmental delay. History shows us that it was and still is very hard to prove the cause of Autism. Even today, they cannot prove the genetic factor as solid evidence as some doctors claim. However, the facts of history and some the information in this book will draw a more positive conclusion on the children that are born normally, years later to contract the disease. In the early years, when these prominent rich families were in denial of their children's autism, they quickly assumed that maybe autism was contagious, maybe it was something the child may have touched, making the environmental theory until this day.

However, that was ruled out later years by many families. History's parents were puzzled to see one of their own children with autism knowing that no one in their family history ever contracted the illness. Cases in point, today many families that have an autism child, do not have autism in their family history; neither do I. There was more money to be made on this growing problem and many researchers and doctors joined the cause. Doctors today have called this other type of Autism apart from the norm due to the "environmental factors" we live with today, as some in history thought it may have been.

However, this is a theory that could never be proven. They say it could have been genetically caused, but in actuality they just do not know! Today they are trying to be so convincing to the public using these excuses, but is a very argumentative issue. The medical community has even added street drugs to their theories, apart from the environmental factors, as a reason for the development of Autism. It seems over the years they've been adding more reasons to the list as to why a child is diagnosed with Autism years after birth. Even parents have hit the list of reasons as being unfit parents to this dilemma. The medical community can assume what they want because they are allowed to, and it is their job to protect their reputations, their interests, and their crimes against over excessive antibiotics on our children.. What I have a problem with is the medical community, doctors, and our own Governmental Health Department ignoring the cries of parents in the 1980s.

Parents, complaining of their children's Autism due to the Amoxicillin doctors were administering to their children; then as time went by their children contracted the Autism Affect. Today those children are about 40 years of age suffering the challenges of life, trying to fit in, trying to live a productive life, being outcasts by many ignorant neighbors, plus an uneducated society regarding what autism is. The fact that this government could have done something about Amoxicillin 30 years ago really breaks me apart.

This was back in the 1980s, and parents were laughed at and ignored by the medical community. When you have parents living in different places in this country, parents that do not know each other, and they all arrive at the same conclusion: that indeed their children started to develop autism after tlong regiments of Amoxicillin, what does that say about Amoxicillin back then in the 1980s Think about what is going on here long and hard. These are facts I am giving you. Could today's production of Autism on our babies have been prevented if some action had taken place against the accuse antibiotic Amoxicillin in the 1980s? I say yes! In addition, this is a question that will be answered in your mind and in your heart by the time you finish reading this book. I hope so. What does that say about our Government of the 1980s who heard the cries of these families and did not come to their rescue? Just like in my case, I cried out to our government about what they did to my grandbaby. They completely ignored me just the same.

After my research I find that the medical community wore down the families of the 1980s with how wrong they were about Amoxicillin. With excuses of genetic and environmental possibilities, it was a perfect brainwash operation of excuses of the 1980s epidemic of Autism caused by Amoxicillin in this country. In the 1980s Amoxicillin was still in the introduction stage to all family clinics and pediatricians. It was their new drug for all pediatric clinics in the country.

The 1980s was the time when the Amoxicillin antibiotic was so well advertised that it became the #1 antibiotic for children and families, which knocked down all other antibiotics that were used by all clinics in this country as time passed, even the placebo. Amoxicillin took over in the 1980s for our children's ear infections and other ailments – understood not to damage children's health. Incredibly, after 30 years, today Amoxicillin is free, and in some stores at the lowest price ever - only $4.00 a cycle, and it is the #1 recommended antibiotic for our children as they planned it to be thirty years ago. In the 1980s the pharmaceutical companies were not about to let anything or anyone stand in the way of their objectives of amoxicillin for babies and children and families. Of course, they have done just that by ignoring the concerns of families about amoxicillin. However, today is a new day with a wake up call for all families. These masterminds have managed to deal with and program any attack against their # 1 antibiotic Amoxicillin, by using tactics that would work against anyone that would even try to knock the drug down.

In this country, we have a right under our Constitution to voice our opinions and concerns, most of all information that can help our children, our people. Do not be afraid of the opposition, pharmaceutical companies who could care less about you or your families. We have the right to warn others, regardless. After learning the truth, you should get the word out to your loved ones, to your neighbors, to your daughters. We must save as many children as possible by spreading the message the old fashioned way - word of mouth spreads faster than imagined.

I gave you solid information about our history on the subject, and the birth of Amoxicillin, and the torture of my baby. Some of you, however, will refuse to see the truth even after you have heard my baby's story of torture, pain, blood, sweat and tears that led to the diagnosis of his Autism today. This is a torture that is being performed every day on our children.

Some of you will stand your ground, claiming that I need more proof, because you hold your profession in medicine and will not make that claim against Amoxicillin. Maybe you just like to be objective. Frankly, my concern is to save as many children as I can from this pharmaceutical amoxicillin web of destruction against our children. You doctors and brown nosing followers out there, even knowing deep inside that you people are wrong, you will still stand firm and disagree.

That is to be expected from most of you. However, for the logical-minded people, families of today and the families of the 1980s, your disapproval is to be commended. We Americans are used to hearing objections to the truth, of important matters in our courts and society today, which we the people have lived on government lies for centuries. Again, whichever way you want to slice it - the evidence is here is in front of you. All you have to do is follow the trail of evidence and deceit, and put the dots together to be able to see the facts regarding why Autism strikes 1 in 88. Look at the history, look at the 1900s, 1970, 1980, 2006, 2008, 2009 and put it all together.

For the skeptically minded people, you are welcome to do your own studies and research on the subject, and for the medical community - No More Lies! It may be a fact that Amoxicillin kills infection, and that an adult can handle many cycles of Amoxicillin given to us in long periods because our bodies can handle it. However, it is also a fact that this drug has ruined the lives of hundreds of thousands of infants and children in this country and abroad, with Rotor Virus and many other viruses caused by over excessive amoxicillin, you know too well. It has even caused the death of babies in this country and abroad... These deaths of our babies, plus harming our children's development are uncalled for. This tragedy must end, and you the families of America can put an end to this growing horror. They have better drugs that can be used without harming our children; you do not have to believe me - do your research!

The question is to whom do they give the better drug to? To only families of stature, maybe? Maybe, the next time you would ask your pediatrician, to recommend a much better drug than the one she is recommending. Let us not forget our history with our parents who used home remedies, herbs, spices, garlic, for our ailments and infections, remedies that can be found on the Internet, you can never deny that. Parents, it's time to put our foot down for our children and ourselves.

One can only imagine why pediatricians don't tell you the truth about the danger level when it comes to your baby using Amoxicillin many times in the past. I am not talking about side effects but the danger affects. Maybe they are too busy to realize it. Maybe they are blinded by success and cannot see what is happening to our children and Amoxicillin. Maybe it's a profit game? There are a lot of maybes here, and you cannot blame me for feeling this way!

Please do not insult my intelligence - I am not criticizing your pediatricians who have done caring, wonderful work with our children. I am talking about a system—a system created to produce results in all categories. But in the category of our children, the amoxicillin system does not work because it damages the child internally in a short time period, harming the child's intestinal tract, building spoors of bacteria that will affect the child's mind in a time period. In my opinion, in reality this is an attack on our children for money - nothing else!

We as a people must call for an end of Amoxicillin and our children. Look again at what has happened during the pass thirty years - 1 in 88 children. We cannot say why the medical community has allowed this to happen to our children; we can only wonder at all possibilities. For me, its is a legalized crime against our children with amoxicillin, as you will see no laws have been broken here—all treatments are legal. Pediatricians should know this danger exists for our children, or maybe they do not know.

Fact is, the Amoxicillin destruction on our babies is happening right in front of them, and this story should be a wake-up call for all pediatricians alike. Again, I remind you, when it comes to a child that is born with Autism, there is no question at its birth of autism, because the baby's system has been compromised along with other organs at birth due to circumstances. However, there is another type of Autism that is created not from birth, but which occurs in later years after so much intake of the antibiotic of first choice called Amoxicillin. It is affecting our children day after day, year after year prescribed by pediatricians and administered by the parent all over the United States. Amoxicillin can cause permanent developmental delay and other difficulties to most children that are exposed to the antibiotic on more than one regimen, and lengthy cycles of Amoxicillin.

Amoxicillin is needlessly used beyond control especially on babies and children. Over-medicating your child is just adding more problems to come.

You know, it is a blessing that we have doctors in this country to cure the sick. It's a shame we have doctors in this country that are nothing but deceitful liars, thieves on insurance, and some that could not care if you die because you have no money or insurance. However, we do have good doctors in America who would tell you not to ever use Amoxicillin on your child. In addition, there are doctors that would tell you that Amoxicillin is safe for your child, and the question is "which one is right?"

The doctors on the right - or - the doctors on the left? Question is - Why can't both have the same opinions? There is a big problem in this country, the rich man dies and leaves a will, and the poor man dies and leaves a bill, remember that. It is not what you know, but who you know to get ahead. To each his own is today's philosophy in this country. But my philosophy is that the truth will set you free, and no matter how powerful one may think he is – there is always room for truth. The real information has been covered up far too long, blinding the families of America on what is really going on with Amoxicillin and children. The strategy they have used over the years in continuing to use Amoxicillin for ear infections on babies has been working in their favor financially, with no interruptions. They can go back to the drawing board and create a better antibiotic, one that will not damage our children's immune system or interfere with our children's vital organs. It really bothers me when a person feels in his heart that he has found an answer to a growing problem, but he would keep it to himself because he feels that friends or his peers may ridicule him.

He doesn't realize the help he could have given to millions of people. This is what I am doing here: Take it! I know how hard it must have been for some families in the 1980s that knew Amoxicillin caused their children's developmental delay, and were probably afraid to continue the fight after they were put down on how wrong they were. For me the complaint of the families of the 1980s was correct, and it is they who are heroes. When a person learns about something that can help our children and families of America, spit it out, let them know what is going on.

You are our children's only hope and prayer for a better tomorrow, and you do not have to be a doctor, a professor, a scholar, but just a regular person who cares that can make a difference, and I intend to do just that. Do not be afraid of telling it like it is, after all, there are people who would stand by you because you care. This is what it took for me to tell the truth that almost took the life of my grandbaby, that changed his life forever……

15
HISTORY OF AUTISM

The discovery of Autism goes back as far as the early 1900s, and is assumed to go back possibly as far as hundreds of years. In 1911, a Swiss Psychiatrist named Eugene Blueler gave Autism its name. He did not quite understand the illness by way of physical appearance and the tendencies of non-communicative behavior, so he classified the term autism as adult schizophrenia.

Through time, it became more apparent and unbelievable that autism was applied more on children of stature, not the children from lower economic strata's. Therefore, doctors were given the challenge to try to find an answer to the cause of autism because it hit people of stature primarily and not the lower class.

In 1943 a doctor from Johns Hopkins University, Dr. Leo Kanner, for the first time put a description on autism by observing 11 children who had withdrawal from human contact from the age of 1 year old. He conducted this test from 1938 to 1943. He noticed the common traits among the children's impairments in social interaction and the anguish they displayed regarding changes because they hated changes in routine. They had a very good memory, belated echolalia, over sensitivity to certain stimuli especially with sound, food problems, and limitations in spontaneous activity especially with others. They had good intellectual potential depending on family background, because it was noticed that talented families of college backgrounds were among the many with children being diagnosed with Autism; therefore, he called the children Autistic. In 1944, Hans Asperger, independent of Leo Kanner, wrote about a group of children he called autistic psychopaths.

In these days if a doctor was to give that description to an autism child his reputation would be destroyed, not to mention he would also find himself in court over a lawsuit. In most cases, they resembled the children of Dr. Kenner's description, the difference was that Hans did not mention echolalia (repetition of words) as a linguistic problem, but the children talked like little grown-ups. Makes you wonder about our children of today with Autism, who typically cannot talk at all until they reach later years.

My baby did not talk until he was 4 years old due to the amount of bacteria that disrupted his system. In addition to Hans, he mentioned their motor activity, which was more clumsy and different from that of a normal child. Bruno Bettelheim wrote about three sessions with children. He called it - "The Empty Fortress." In his writings, he too called the children Autistic, but he claimed that their disorder was due to the coldness of their mothers. He totally disengaged the parents from the children's therapy and consistently putting more weight on the parents as the cause of the problem, which I think was crazy of him. Back then, they did not respect women as they do today; they treated women horribly in those days and it's no wonder that the parents would take the blame. Until this day the parents have always gotten the blame. Of course this man, Bruno Bettelheim, and some of his writings against mothers were not to be respected. Authorities realized later that mothers had nothing to do with the cause of Autism.

For the children that are diagnosed with Autism Spectrum Disorders in later years, doctors all over since the beginning have tried to pinpoint the problem. Doctors and researchers today cannot truly say that it was street drugs or environmental factors that caused these children to have Autism, because it did not make any sense to the researchers and doctors in those years, even today.

Many know that excessive Amoxicillin is causing the rising numbers of children being diagnosed with Autism due to contaminating the child's system.

But we cannot get past the power of pharmaceutical companies controlling their product. It is all about money and power. During the 1940s through the 1960s the medical community felt that children who had Autism where Schizophrenic. This lack of understanding of Autism Disorder and the history led many parents to think that maybe it was their fault, and of course some doctors agreed, covering up the truth of the matter. Since the beginning for hundred years, the blame was always somewhat directed toward the parents. They just could not understand how and why Autism was created, so they looked for a scapegoat to blame it on like the parents to protect themselves and their reputation in the medical community from looking incompetent for some answers. This is what was told to me by a retired doctor living in my neighborhood. With the knowledge of Autism, we can see the parents are and have been victims of circumstance for one hundred years.

What history has shown us during the 1960s was that people began to understand Autistic behavior. More importantly, they began to identify autistic symptoms and treatments. However, today we see some doctors along the way starting to change what we have learned about Autism. They would assume street drugs, genes, environmental to be the cause, but I tell you a victory is still in the making. The work of Hans Asperger with Autism did not become known until the end of the 1980s.

That's when his book was translated into English. Kanner and Bettelheim's works were quite often confused, and it was generally accepted that autistic children had frigid mothers. In the 1970s knowledge of Autism spread like wildfire in Sweden. The Erica Foundation started education and therapy for psychotic children in the beginning of the 80s, with understanding that Autism was not really a psychotic problem. The first Autistic classes within special education started in the middle of the 1970s. For a very long time Autism and Psychosis continued to be confused, and until this day, parents are accused of causing the serious disabilities their Autistic child has. Moreover, this blame has to end because, in my opinion, parents get the blame so doctors can hide the truth. For many years, researchers searched for the underlying cause of contact and language disorders, but they realized that the disability was more complex than imagined; there was no single basic cause. The bottom line is that no one really knows for sure what causes children to be *born* with Autism.

However, Autism after a normal birth is the big question on everybody's mind. Moreover, on the other end of our current century, children are being diagnosed as time passes. Today we are learning as to why this is. There is no problem understanding; it's more a matter of putting the dots together. All you have to do is look at our history of autism and compare it to today's autism events, and all the Amoxicillin antibiotics that are going into our children.

Just ask yourselves - why was Autism early in the 1900s upon people of stature only, not the poor people or emigrants that came to this country by the thousands on ships, or the native Americans all of whom were not rich or wealthy; why not their children? Again, most experts of today, not from yesteryear's studies would say that probably Autism is caused by a combination of genes and environmental factors, which I do not agree with. I would agree that you can be born with Autism, but to catch Autism after a normal birth coming from a family that never had Autism genetically - well, those experts need to go back to the drawing board and consider the possibilities of Amoxicillin with the track record and research enclosed. Parents do not need to be experts in the medical field to know their own child's behavior and where it came from, and how their child received Autism coming from a normal childbirth. In the 1980s autism research accelerated, and more and more researchers joined the bandwagon and became convinced that the basic reasons were to be found in neurological disturbances.

Of course, in my opinion more doctors joined the bandwagon in the 1980s because of all the complaints about the Amoxicillin Autism Affect from families. Some experts say the cause is sometimes combined with hereditary illnesses, such as PKU or chromosomal aberrations such as fragile X-chromosome would be examples. Of course, this makes sense but what about the families that reject that notion? There was so much different research being done in spite of the multitude of causes for Autism that they claimed, there were similarities that made it possible to group these children under the same diagnosis.

It was also observed that the autistic children among themselves were very different in many ways. There was a whole spectrum, from severely retarded multi-handicapped children to extreme gifted eccentrics. Instead of just talking autism, they started to talk of Autism Spectrum Disorders (Plural). Today a wide umbrella of many disorders, developed years after a normal birth is what has been going on for the past 30 years and this development of Autism is my argument.

For me it is self-explanatory when looking at the history of events and today's current events on the subject is what is really going on here. According to the American Academy of Pediatrics (AAP), autism is not a specific disease, but rather a collection of disorders of brain development called "Autism Spectrum Disorders" or ASDs. Autism does not require having a collection of disorders in order to recognize one has the Autism.

Some with autism spectrum disorder may have the ability to do certain things better than the normal child, while other children with Autism may not have the ability to understand concepts. Some Autistic children may not like athletics, while others do. The American Academy of Pediatrics also says that autism has a strong genetic basis. While they may be searching for more facts on the birth of Autism, many cases show interest in the creation of Autism, as I am. One of the questions of this book is, "Can autism be created by medicine, especially Amoxicillin?"

You can assume autism is a genetic based creation; other doctors would argue they find it difficult to prove that Autism comes from vaccines, environmental or genetics unless a twin is involved. We see many cases to show no relatives have had Autism in their family history, unless of course there is a neurological problem in family history; but it dose not count for the vast increase of Autism the pass Ten Years as such for Genes. Although there may be a case in which you may find a gene connection or something else, it does not speak for the population. Studies show that the development of autism has risen in the past 30 years tremendously. It's no wonder you have many differences of opinion on the subject; everybody wants to be a hero. I have a problem with the introduction of Amoxicillin in the 1970s and the 1980s into a widespread use in all the clinics in America. Besides all the explanations, the apparent increase in autism also may be due to a combination of factors we don't hear about every day.

For example, more and more behaviors and disorders are being identified and included in the definition of Autism Spectrum Disorders than in past history. The identifications help gather these children so they are not left behind in the services they need. If they do not receive services, many will grow into a world of confusion or even crime. The public and the medical professionals recognize these disorders more often today than ever before. I admire the American Academy of Pediatrics for their hard work for these children, and I like the way they tell pediatricians that early diagnosis of these children is crucial.

Unfortunately, not all pediatricians heed what AAP has to say about early diagnosis, because I know that there are pediatricians who tell parents who complain about their babies behavior that "all kids are like that; let's wait till the baby is 3 or 4 years old to see what happens, then we'll test them." This is what pediatricians say on more than one occasion to concern parents about early detection. I also like the way AAP tells pediatricians to listen carefully to the parents about their child's development. Briefly, for any doctor to put a genetic assessment on a child for their Autism Spectrum Disorder without looking at the whole picture of family history and doing an in depth research on children, it is unprofessional. We have a multi high rise of Autistic children who are diagnosed years after birth, unlike the child that was born with developmental problems to assume it may be genetic by looking into the family medical history. This group is different. Parents are saying "yes" we have members in our family who have autism, or "no" we don't have family members with autism.

Of course, the ones that are diagnosed with autism in the later years after a normal birth are said to contract the disease from environmental factors or genetics. However, positive research has shown and some doctors also feel is that the majority from the environmental factors, as assumed by the medical community, have been ruled out. Countless parents from the 1980s and up to today, (including myself) see that excuse as ridiculous as the Air Force telling us it was a weather balloon and not a UFO.

That is leaving thousands of parents unanswered regarding their children's autism, and parents convincing themselves there is no other explanation, so it must be environmental or genetic; *Someone in my family may have had it, we don't know? Forget About It!*

Many parents agree, including me, that our children's autism is a result of the antibiotic Amoxicillin we administered to our children. The evidence of my grandson with 34 cycles in nine months leads to the conclusion of the source for many children.. There have been many theories discussed but the cause or causes of autism of the vast increase are still not known from birth - we all know that. However, an in-depth study should be done on antibiotics in connection to autism, if I am correct. More research is being done every year to try to identify the causes and improve efforts to prevent incorrect diagnoses, and to treat ASD, but nothing is being done on this research in question of the amoxicillin autism affect. The AAP says the nation's top experts in pediatric neurology, genetics, and other fields are moving closer to answers about this group of disorders.

This brings me to say that it's the parents who have to recognize these disorders more and more, and share their findings with the medical professionals." In turn, the professionals must record their findings that the AAP is trying to get credit for. In the eyes of the professionals, parents are secondary to the achievements of their sick children, and frankly, I am tired of seeing it! Tired of hearing it! I would like AAP and doctors abroad to understand that those working for some answers on how their children caught the Autism disease are the world's top experts themselves-"The Parents!"

The parents are the professionals. The American Academy of Pediatrics is dedicated to the health of all children and we are ever so grateful to have them, but let us not forget that the parents are truly the world's leading experts. They know their child better than any doctor, something the AAP should always remember when speaking of 'experts with children.' Parents never get credit, and I credit them! More researchers say Autism is what they call *innate*. Innate is a contact disorder. Normally, infants early after birth orient themselves toward the human face and voice, and response to voices and facial expression. However, autistic children cannot interpret another person's face and do not imitate as automatically. This is the reason why later in life they are not able to share attention and experiences with others because of the innate disorder. Many experiences would be missed that way. The basis of socialization is to contact and imitate.

The autistics have difficulty in seeing another person's perspective, in understanding the thoughts and intentions of others. There are researchers who believe the basic cause of this is a difficulty in shifting attention. The same attention shifting difficulty would also lead to the ritualistic behaviors and the difficulties in managing change, difficulty in interrupting one activity, and changing to another.

OTHER SIGNS PARENTS SHOULD NOTICE AS FOLLOWS -

Central Coherence - Does not automatically look for the meaning of what is going on. Detailed vision - The world consists of isolated details and not a coherent inner map. Processing information one piece at a time - Has difficulties with information consisting of several parts.

The autistic also have difficulties with void time when nothing happens as well as changing from one activity to another. These are just some important noticeable expressions of concern for parents to make note of in infants early after birth. Do not wait until years pass to find out that the child has autism. There are many indicators based on observation comparing a normal child with the autistic child. Parents can reach out to their pediatricians or

Children's Medical Services, which they have in most areas where parents live. They will share with the parent what signs to look for, but we as parents can easily recognize what has changed along the way for our baby and children, especially if your baby or children have been on Amoxicillin regimens.

Remember the indicator for us grandparents, parents, guardians, babysitters, preschool teachers, is to focus on developmental viewing of your baby and children around you. It's a gift we are born with to be able to recognize everything in front of us, and it's time for us to use it and mass-produce that gift for the benefit of our children. Please do not wait until the child is four or five years old before you take a good look at your child's behavioral characteristics.

We should not feel guilty for not realizing the warning signs; life has been hard for the most part. However, there should be no excuse from now on because we realize them now, and how important it is for our baby's future, because I know you truly love your baby, and this is your wake up call!

16
TAKE AMOXICILLIN OUT

We have learned so far, doctors and pediatricians who may or may not know the truth behind it all will not confirm that Amoxicillin can cause another form of Autism and Developmental Delay on a child. We know that Autism can be easily caused by excessive and long-term antibiotic treatments on infants and children. For years people have been claiming vaccines can give our children Autism.

Of course, there was a time when families accused Penicillin for the Autism Affect. Moreover, in other case studies they found amounts of mercury in children with Autism, with convincing evidence that the amount of mercury was causing destruction to the immune system and the mind.

Having an affect of Developmental Delay problems, but it does not explain the vast increase of autism we see today, and parents do not exercise using Penicillin any longer. The antibiotic that has been in the spotlight, and ignored by the medical community, is Amoxicillin and Augmentin. Many parents feel this drug indeed has cause many children to contract the Autism disease affect, as described by myself and other parents testimonies, disputed by the medical community it cannot be. Today Penicillin is rarely used or accepted by many families' even pediatricians, for the same destruction amoxicillin is causing our children today. However, amoxicillin is still on active duty for children in America. All these cases are public information. All antibiotics related to amoxicillin we hear about also have been added to the cause of the Amoxicillin Autism Affect.

The big factor here is when you administer antibiotics to your baby, you are adding a substance that in later time may interfere with the child's development for a productive life, and you will never know that unless your pediatrician explains the danger level of the antibiotic that your child has been taking since birth. If you have been giving your baby this medicine, you will be there to witness your baby's developmental changes in a few years, if you continue on the same medicine for most of your children's illnesses.

There are a great many stories you can read about in your Google search, just as you are hearing about my baby right now. The families of the 80s and my grandson's case, along with many other complaints about amoxicillin, my friends, is your living proof of this problem we are facing today among our children. You must stop and think - Ask yourselves, – "What about all those people who have been complaining all these years of their children's Autism caused by Amoxicillin? - Are they crazy? Am I crazy?" I do not think so! What about the 34 cycles in 9 months of amoxicillin given to my grandbaby over an ear infection ordered by the doctor? Is the doctor crazy? I think so! Am I crazy for following the doctors' orders? I think so! Put the puzzle together, my friends. We have been programmed to follow the direction of this continuing problem upon our children. We lack training or experience with medications because we are used to believing and trusting our medical doctors. The medical authorities in this country will tell you that all families that have their Autistic Children and link the problem to Amoxicillin are all false.

They say this to us because they are the professionals on the subject and know you will follow their recommendations. We follow and obey their explanations, because we do not trust ourselves to seek the right answers—because we've been conditioned to place our trust in them. This is how our human minds have been operating, under their control of blindsiding the reality of what has been going on with our children being diagnosed with Developmental Delay Autism.

For thirty years since the introduction of Amoxicillin, we have been destroying our babies' immune systems faster with this deadly medicine. It's causing our children's diagnoses of Autism today. I do not believe a vaccine comprises a major cause, as I said earlier. If that were true that vaccines cause Autism, then my wife, my children, most Americans and maybe even the President like I said earlier, would have had some type of autism, because of the vaccines we had to take as children. Moreover, the vast increase of children being diagnose with autism today would be - 1 in 5 children. Then by some miracle over the years my autism and everyone else's magically went away; I do not think so! What I do think, is that some parents attack the vaccines their children have taken as a cause of their children's Autism because they have no other answer as to why their child has Autism. They don't know or realize that all the while through the years, they have been harming the child's insides, their system.

They're giving their children antibiotics such amoxicillin for ear infections and other sicknesses, with doctors orders. At the same time they were thinking in their minds - if their pediatrician was giving their babies Amoxicillin it must be safe; not realizing the pediatrician by-pass the 20 cycles danger level for the child, this of course is a major problem in this country with pediatricians. They think in their minds that the antibiotic just flushes out of the baby's system when the baby does potty.

I spoke to many parents, and it seems that some parents feel that the Amoxicillin simply flushes out of the baby's system, that its safe as said by their pediatrician. This, of course, has me wondering about the pediatricians that they do not take time to explain these things. Therefore, to the parent it has to be the vaccine that caused their child's Autism because that is the only answer they can think of. This way of thinking is not stupid, it is just innocence because parents do not know the history of the repercussions of Amoxicillin today or in past history, what it does to their baby's immune system and vital organs, especially in infants. I have been explaining an unforeseen problem that has destroyed many children and families in our time and history even to many babies' death. The one drug that has been in the spotlight for many parents for thirty years, have been ignored by our government, the news media, and the medical community on the subject of amoxicillin. I cannot understand or comprehend why and who was the mastermind behind making this antibiotic Amoxicillin the # 1 medicine for ear infections and other ailments on our children after all the damage it can cause.

With major complaints from parents until this day in time— indeed, after the complaints in the 1980s, these pharmaceutical companies back then that knew of the allegations of Amoxicillin should have stopped the selling of this drug. The heroes in my journey of discovery are my grandson Chris for hanging on to life, and the families of the 1980s for stepping up to the plate against amoxicillin.

Unless they conduct an in-depth study on all the families with autistic children making a claim against Amoxicillin you will never know the solid truth about Amoxicillin, and frankly, they would never allow such a study. You can however believe what I say here is truth, facts do not lie, and the study is here. These families from the 1980s would be the best subjects for this study, because indeed Amoxicillin caused their children's Autism, which I truly believe today. The pharmaceutical company that is reading this book about these allegations of Amoxicillin and Autism - for them it's old news, because they remember what happened in the 1980s. The medical community ignored parents' complaints over Amoxicillin causing their children's Autism. The pharmaceutical companies and doctors felt that the parent or caregiver was at fault here for their children's disorders, not the Amoxicillin. After what happened to my grandbaby, I know the Amoxicillin Autism Affect is real and is not going away. The medical community has many excuses when it comes to this subject. The irony of this, is that Amoxicillin does not work on ear infections.

It works on the disruption of the baby's growth. It ruins your insides, your immune system, intestines, digestive tract, then the affects start to take hold. Repeated doctor visits for Amoxicillin for the baby is a reality in every clinic in America; this is crossing the line. Doctors must set their tactics in making profit gains on another category from patients, and not on babies. The 1980s was a time of struggle for these parents because they felt defeated by their own government against what was happening to their children over Amoxicillin.

As time passed on, so did life continue to pass on? So this is a subject that has remained in the file cabinet for 30 years. Nevertheless, I am here to pull the file out of the cabinet thirty years later. It's time to let the truth out of the cabinet to dispute these negative doctors on the subject that indeed the Amoxicillin Autism Affect is real, and is here to stay. There are doctors and researchers who feel Amoxicillin surely does cause Developmental Delay Autism, just like what happened to my baby. I have quoted the good doctors in this book who have conducted their own research. They outlined that, indeed, Amoxicillin is another leading cause of developmental delay and Autism if used excessively over the duration period of the drug, passing the cycle point of danger with no return. Unfortunately, doctors have been doing just that as it reads.

Look over your shoulder and ask the first mother you see or your sister or relatives whether their baby has been sick in the past with an ear infection or something else, then ask them about the cycles of Amoxicillin that were administered to the baby from their pediatrician, and see what those parents have to say. It is a growing problem, my friends. Too many cycles would be lethal and deadly and pediatricians know this to be true.

Many children have died already over Amoxicillin, and the parent is pointed out for the blame, or Amoxicillin as a cause in the death of a child is described as a terrible mistake.

The misuse and over excessive Amoxicillin antibiotic treatments will create a bacterium in the baby's immune system unseen, of course, to the naked eye. Other internal organs will affect their brains as time passes finally resulting in the disruption of the baby's neurotransmitters in their brains. These disruptions automatically cause Developmental Delay within a period of so many cycles of their # 1 drug, Amoxicillin, given to that baby. This, of course, would only occur if they survive the excessive Amoxicillin treatments administered in the child's lifetime. Many children have died from the creation of bacterium C-Difficile, B Toxin, and Rotavirus. The buildup of bacteria will get so toxic in the immune system, the intestinal tract, the digestive tract, and then in time he will be diagnosed with Autism and many spectrum disorders. When this diagnosis of Autism occurs for the child, then, unbelievably from pass history till this day pediatricians blame it on genetics or environmental factors, and the parent, of course. The Amoxicillin Autism Affect has been with us and ignored for thirty years.

Now is time for honesty to kick in about the damage this is wreaking on our children's development for the rest of their lives. For the moment let us put aside the doctors' reasoning that the child can get C-Difficile bacteria by touching or not washing their hands. Even though the child can pick up some type of virus by not washing their hands or by touching something, I ask that you try to see the clear picture here. Please do not misunderstand; I am grateful for Amoxicillin saving countless lives from deadly infections.

My concern is the build-up of deadly infectious bacteria in the baby's immune system, intestines, digestive tract, caused by the excessive Amoxicillin treatments that pediatricians have exercised in this country. If your child ever gets really sick, with diarrhea, vomiting, loss of appetite, losing weight—then have his stool tested and his blood for infectious bacteria in his system, and find out how many cycles your child has taken of Amoxicillin in your child's history from your pediatricians or pharmacist.

Our children get ear infections that can be cured with ear tubes to drain out the fluids. Runny noses, fever, respiratory problems - all that can be cured with other options instead of Amoxicillin in all cases. There is a great margin in the administration of antibiotics to our kids and it has to be addressed. It's simple, really. Amoxicillin has its advantages in saving lives, but has its disadvantages hurting, destroying, and changing the developmental life of a baby and a child forever. The Autism will be noticed when the child starts going to school.

Remember, these are our children and we must go the extra mile for their safety and security so they can live a productive life. No doctor has the right to try an experiment on a baby or child in an attempt to cure an ear infection after knowing all the side affects and the dangers of the drug. The danger can alter a child's immune system, intestinal tract, which is a leading cause of developmental problems for the baby or child. This information should be exposed and advertised throughout this nation— reason why I am writing this book.

A child with developmental delay did not ask for this disability after being born normal. Either the child is born with a disability, or the disability was placed there through a timeline of disruption within the child's system with infectious bacteria. Hundreds of thousands of Autistic Children here in America that are born normal, are later diagnosed as autistic. For a doctor to do Amoxicillin experiments on a child, even over an ear infection instead of using ear tubes, knowing what that baby may go through the rest of the baby's life with the build-up of internal infectious bacteria, I say that doctor is crazy. That is putting it mildly; these doctors should be stripped of their medical license, knowing the overview. This is a crazy way of life causing Autism and Developmental Delay from the antibiotics given to our children in this country in the name of experimentation.

It's actually in the name of money and profits; that is how I feel! This type of Amoxicillin Autism Affect is far less different from full-blown Autism that your baby may be born with at birth. My heart goes out to children with this Autism Affect. Some children will remain more serious than others who contract the disease after a normal birth. These children will reflect low functioning at first, and maybe high functioning later on in life, and will experience confusion for the rest of their lives. Their social skills, their motor skills, their communication skills and learning abilities - all will be affected today and in their future.

When a child is infected with this disease the child tries to be constructive with himself half the time, he is having unwanted meltdowns most of the time, and is being misunderstood by his peers and the school system. The

Amoxicillin Autism Affect is the other Autism apart from the natural Autism that you are born with. Your immune system and the brain are already compromised at birth. The Autistic child at birth is more visible to the eye, but the Autism that is diagnosed in later years—-these children are misunderstood even with a special direction for education and survival. In regard to these children who are diagnosed after a normal birth, they will be a little different to handle, being that they lived a normal life for 3 to 5 years before being diagnosed with Autism. Society today labels some medical problems more credible than others, and, of course, the more credible they are considered the most services they will receive.

An individual educational plan for the child's education and future is gratefully appreciated from all parents. These children are in the middle of low functioning and high functioning. For the Autistic after a normal birth a new alteration takes place in the development of the child. Their neurotransmitters are not quite connected in proper form, the way they were when they were born normal. Something happened between birth and 5 years later, and most of times he would not know if he is coming or going, making it harder on the parents and educators to understand his needs.

At times, a teacher may look at the functionally autistic and feel that he is just a normal child. In time, the teacher will come to realize that indeed her student is an autistic child. It is without question that both the child that is Autistic at birth, and the child that is infected with the Amoxicillin Autism Affect will always be special needy children that would need love and care 24 hours a day, 7 days a week with a special heart to bear.

They both would have different disorders but always in the same direction. My anger stretches from thousands of families from past history until today who felt back then that Amoxicillin was the cause for the Amoxicillin Autism Affect on their child. Not one health official in our government cared to do anything about it, not even an investigation in the 1980s. The medical community professionals themselves, by allowing Amoxicillin to contaminate our babies with too many cycles in the baby's system, have caused the autism affect.

It is the making of this type of Autism that has been hidden in the closet for 30 years, and the medical community knows about the affects of Amoxicillin and the baby's system. I know a family, discovers that their child developed the Amoxicillin Autism Affect. Their child's pediatricians recorded their findings as a genetic affect or environmental affect on the child, and not what the parent said, that she felt it was the amoxicillin.

But on the patient's medical records it does not show the parent mentioning the amoxicillin consumption. This is a regular practice for doctors today, ignoring the parent's knowledge of what is happening to their child. Always protecting them from the Amoxicillin complaint that is destroying our children. Moreover, families today continue to use Amoxicillin on their babies because of the trust they have in their baby's doctor's recommendations.

Parents do not want to see their babies crying in pain but little they know there are other methods and other medications less dangerous for their child's ear infections, throat infections and so on—even home remedies. Many families do not research the probability that the Amoxicillin they have been administering to their child could be the cause for their child's developmental problems. We must face the truth that some doctors are not truthful with us!

In addition, what gets me is that some doctors are blindsided themselves. Some doctors and pediatricians do not realize what they are doing to the baby's system will affect them for the rest of the baby's life when constant cycles Amoxicillin is being administered into the baby's system. Some of these doctors do not take the time to do research on the antibiotic that they administer to the baby. They follow recommendations from the pharmaceutical representatives.

The problem there is that these doctors should already have been informed by doing their own research of what is truly going on between Amoxicillin and children. They should do their own research on the medicines that they prescribe to children instead of relying on a sales representative's direction on the drug. How these doctors over-medicate our babies is incomprehensible.

In my opinion, they do this because they know you will return, with the babies developing more health problems that Amoxicillin is causing inside their small bodies, contaminating the baby's system. Again, there's allot of maybes here, and I just do not understand. This is a country divided with a slogan saying - "To Each His Own." There are few caring hearts for children and families when it comes to this topic of Amoxicillin and autism. You must put your foot down and always be on top of things when it comes to your baby, and be your baby's own doctor. Doctors should take the time to find out more about the amoxicillin they give our children; instead pediatricians listen to the professional sales representatives from pharmaceutical companies that are selling the drug, bypassing the most dangerous probability of injury toward our children. What is the reality here?

Another thing that passed by me for years is that most of the time you go into a clinic with your baby, it seems more concern is evident regarding the insurance that pays the bill than your baby's health. This is a fact; just ask other parents about it. This should be a red flag for all families when they go to a doctor that cares more about money than your baby's health. To me, doctors see an unconcerned parent about their children's medication and their baby's internal system, but it's because they trust the doctor.

That is what the doctors sees in the parent when the parent does not have important questions for the doctor, and they know this because they know we trust them. They may have contempt for the baby's ailment just like the parents at the time. The doctor will just give the parent a prescription for Amoxicillin, which will seem satisfactory for them both; but never once, but there is no concern about the history of the baby with that same type of medication (that the baby may have been consuming throughout the months or even years). Now, the doctor makes a follow up appointment to see how the baby has done with the infection and Amoxicillin, continuing treatments on the baby if the baby's infection did not go away; and of course more money is then paid by the insurance. It is a controlled systematic operation to keep that money rolling in.

Easy money; more destruction on the baby. I do not care how much money we may have to pay a doctor for caring for my child the right way, but I do care how the clinic represents itself and the quality healthcare my baby will receive. They love money more than taking care of our children. Hidden by the power of more money, some doctors are blind to the fact of what is really going on here. With so many children in the matter a few years, the multitude of children being diagnosed with Autism and Developmental Delay is a horrifying reality.

Our researchers themselves are confused regarding how these children are catching this disease in an alarming rate. Pharmaceutical companies who make the drug will not heed any red flags connecting amoxicillin and children. What should we do? How long must this go on? After conducting my research, I believe that there are many doctors who truly see the destruction that Amoxicillin is causing our children today. The information is widespread against Amoxicillin from past history, and it is unbelievable that a doctor can be that illiterate not to know this information. I believe the medical community knows that what they did was wrong in making the antibiotic Amoxicillin a wonder drug for babies. I believe also since the people themselves do not care to fight about amoxicillin and our children, or to make enough noise about it; why should they care to do anything? In my opinion, they let this happen, because they have a lot of money to lose if they stop it. I truly believe this is the crazy reason why the medical community has allowed this antibiotic to infect our children all these years since the 1980s.

The equation is here, the missing dots are here. Medical proof with positive research from my boo-boo and studies on amoxicillin are here. The Autism Affect arrived at 1 in 88 today because of past history on Amoxicillin that is disrupting our children's immune system, and the intestinal tract with bacteria that causes developmental problems, the Amoxicillin Autism Affect. You, the readers and parents, will ultimately be the deciding group on this subject regarding what I have described to you, and what I am sharing with you. We have been deceived long enough.

The proper information is denied parents about the true effects of Amoxicillin; instead you receive an explanation of the medicine's side effects when you pick up your prescription on paper. All you have to do is make that extra leap into the record of accomplishment of the Amoxicillin destroying our children. The truth of the matter is that we parents just do not research antibiotics that are given to our children. I never made that extra leap for my grandbaby because I had full confidence and trust in the medical community and the doctors in charge of my baby's ear infection; and they almost killed him! These doctors' did not bother to keep me on my toes about the lengthy excessive Amoxicillin, and the true danger behind it. I had doctors in All Children's Hospital from the emergency room telling me how crazy it was to fill my baby's system with so much Amoxicillin, especially in a nine-month period. They told me the internal disruption and destruction occurred within my baby's system, by allowing the pediatricians to perform the Amoxicillin experiment on an ear infection.

These four pediatricians lied to me about everything. I am not surprised, because we know that this country has lived on lies to run this country, from business owners to doctors, and politicians throughout history upon the people of this country. In my opinion, the pharmaceutical companies that push the antibiotic Amoxicillin drug to doctors, tells them to push the drug on ear infections and throat infections on infants and children, and just about every other ailment the child may have.

They tell these doctors Amoxicillin is a great antibiotic through sale representative's techniques. Techniques are practiced before they leave their office to the field; they are professionals. Millions of children were being infected with infectious bacteria over the years because of this antibiotic Amoxicillin, right underneath our noses. For the many families of the 1980s that got caught in this dilemma, I say to you thank you for your courage and doing your best in this fight.

Do not be discouraged about today's Autism population because this book is the wake up call you all have been waiting for. We victims will not go unheard, and this time the government's Health Department must hear our demands to stop this Amoxicillin Autism Affect, and the mass production we are witnessing today. This is it! As I've repeated many times Amoxicillin and Augmentin are two antibiotics that have been the cause of infectious bacteria in the baby's system causing damage of different proportions to our babies and children over a time period.

Even when they do use the antibiotic the right way, it does not work! The infection comes right back on the child, so what do doctors do? They misuse the drug by forcibly administering excessive treatments on the baby and the children, to see when the drug will take full affect on ear infections and other infections. Adding more cycles than needed of an antibiotic into the baby's system is dangerous, deadly, and permanent. This has been happening right underneath our noses for many years.

We have been blindsided because we were not knowledgeable in these medical areas for our children, and of course, we are always ahead of ourselves, not stopping to evaluate what is in front of us. This is how we live. I have decided to write this book because my grandbaby has suffered the bloodiest Amoxicillin Experiment you can imagine, and today he is Autistic because of it. The guilt on my shoulders is so heavy. I cry every day for not being knowledgeable as a grandfather as I should have been at the time and for following my grandbaby's pediatrician recommendations. My grandbaby's life was almost snuffed out since I was not up to par with the true after-affects of Amoxicillin. At his last almost dying day of my grandbaby before landing in the hospital, his pediatricians would not allow me to take him to an emergency room. I ignored the pediatrician for the first time, and decided to take my baby to the emergency room where they saved his life by one day before his death.

After time passed and I learned the truth of Amoxicillin and children, I knew then that I had to write my grandbaby's story to save as many children as I can in this great country of ours. I see destruction upon our children that we have seen far too long now. You just can't see it on the surface, but you know it's there, and now with a little help you can see it a little clearer. What to do now? May this story inspire all parents to voice your concerns! Write your concerns about Amoxicillin on babies and children that have claimed the death of many babies, and send your letters to President Obama.

Write to the government's Department of Health and to your state governors. If they don't listen let's vote them out of office. For the people of stature in this country that are reading this book like actors and singers, lawyers and scholars. If your children today are suffering Autism or Developmental Delay, and you come to realize that what I'm saying here is the truth, I say to you your voice is strong, and we need your help to stand with us.

If the safety and lives of our children are not important enough for them to hear about Amoxicillin and change laws for our children, why should you donate any money for their campaigns? Why should they be elected? They should be run out of elected office for the people and our children, if they cannot help us against this drug Amoxicillin that is destroying our babies. Together we the people and parents can make a difference; but, divided, our children will continue to fall as they have been for over 30 years on Autism after a normal birth.

In addition, I have a message for the Department of Health that runs this country's children's healthcare: I ask you to listen when it comes to the safety of our children at this time and age. Listen about The Amoxicillin Autism Affect - this is it! Do not even think about treating us as you did the families of the 1980s with complaints of Autism and Amoxicillin that you did not do anything about! Take out Amoxicillin and Augmentin antibiotics out of every clinic in America.

The more parents continue to voice their opinion on this subject, the more attention people and families will draw into our political circle against Amoxicillin. Our government will have to listen to put regulations that would protect our children from excessive antibiotics and making Amoxicillin #1 drug of choice for our children here in America that should have been removed years ago.

Causing internal problems for the baby will automatically make the baby return to their clinic time after time. My opinions and research may sound unwarranted to the medical profession, but the medical profession is not important here. What is important here is the truth of the matter, and this truth is directed to millions of parents. You have to figure out which doctors are telling the truth, and the ones who care for a long-term clean bill of health for our children.

The doctor that makes our children return to his clinic for his profits for a long-term recovery, causing future problems in our children's system and vital organs, will show the affects in later years. Today my grandbaby's autism suffers developmental problems you would not believe, his education and way of life is affected for the rest of his life.

While it is true that is very hard to understand the birth of Autism, it will not be hard for you at all to understand why we have 1 in 88 American children being diagnosed with Autism after you finish reading this book.

This is not rocket science, just hard work putting the puzzle together. It is my belief after doing my research that of 1 in 88 children that are being diagnosed today with autism, these children who have been infected with developmental delay and autism are a result of long-term infectious bacteria building up inside the body in a timeline that will eventually interfere with the brain.

These bacteria are lethal to the baby's immune system, to the intestinal tract, the digestive system; this is what is happening today. This comes through the misuse of Amoxicillin prescribed by pediatricians and medical doctors for years. With government regulations approving such regimens of antibiotics that are given to our children, one can only imagine the work it will take to fix this problem.

I say there is major concern about your baby's development in the next few years if you have been giving your child Amoxicillin all this time. Moreover, there is a major concern over your baby's pediatrician giving your baby so much Amoxicillin even if they say to you - that there is nothing to be concerned about; after all, the government's health department regulates it all. This is unbelievable - but it is all true! You have to observation your child very closely, looking for any slight changes. You have to observe and watch if the baby is doing everything that is normal for the baby's age in time.

It's incredible how so many children are being diagnosed with so many disorders just a few years after birth, something that will affect their future forever. Whether or not pediatricians and doctors deliberately do this Amoxicillin attack on our kids, we will never know. However, we know one thing that doctors should already have known the effects of the drug, and for them to put the responsibility on the parents if something should go haywire, it is wrong and inhuman. It's a question that we parents whose children have been victimized must ask ourselves - are we at fault? Doctors will bear no answer to that question but just look at you as if indeed you are. Through the course of reading this book, many of you will learn the answers to why doctors have allowed this to carry on; all you have to do if you care and want to help is to pass this book and information on to other families. While reading this book, think for a moment, is there someone you know or a family member that this may be happening to right this very moment? Pick up the phone and make that call.

Hinge yourselves on that red flag popping up in your head while you are reading this story. While reading this book if there are any red flags in this story to be recognized as abusive, excessive, and long-term, misdiagnoses, negligence and bloody sadness that you know of, then take action. After you have collected enough of the red flags, after your mind sees the truth, and you see those children in your mind—that's when you can put the complete puzzle together about the hidden truth of the Amoxicillin Autism Affect.

Then you can do something to help yourself, and those you know, and support our cause.

The recipe of 1 in 88 children being infected today for tomorrow's future is right here and you can help stop it. You do not have to be a scholar to put this puzzle together. The Amoxicillin Autism Affect that has been infecting our children and by passing grandparents and parents for thirty years is here, and now you can see and understand, why you have not been able to see how we are harming our children with this junk.

The Amoxicillin Autism Affect is real and is never going away until you make it happen. Many great doctors have foretold the predictions of the danger effects and causing internal damage using Amoxicillin that can cause Developmental Delay and Autism on our babies and children, and now it has happened. This is reality that must not be ignored. Witness for yourselves - do your research.

Top professionals in their field telling the medical community of the damage that over excessive antibiotic have caused our children, some even to their death since the introduction of Amoxicillin. Say a prayer for the millions of families in this country that have not seen justice, for what the medical communities have done to many children including mine. Give this book the power to change the hearts and minds of the medical community. Lets make our voices heard, tell the government and your representitives to - "Take Out Amoxicillin" from every clinic in the Untited States and abroad. Do not ignore the help you can show for all children in America.

17
MAKE NO MISTAKE

Some of you are probably shocked now by what I have shared with you so far. I was shocked myself after learning the truth. An old man said to me once, "When something sounds too good to be true, chances are that it isn't true." He said when something sounds unbelievable it takes only facts to make it believable. That old man was my golf teacher in grammar school many years ago.

I was about to use a three wood from the rough onto the fairway about 200 yards out, with a bunch of trees in my way. He told me to try an unbelievable shot, slice it through a window in the trees to the right toward the green. I said to him that it would be unbelievable that any man can do a shot like that from the rough with a three wood.

He told me that once I calculate the right mathematics I could make that shot believable to the unbeliever. He was a very unusual man in his concepts of golf, and I respected him. I looked, examined, calculated, and believed, especially after I made that shot believable. I made the shot, and it was good. However, I never became Tiger Woods. Reminds me of the challenge that I am up against with all you unbelievers of the Amoxicillin Autism Affect. As beautiful as this country is, it can be very cruel when it comes to healthcare and our Children. This is one of the only free countries in the world without free universal healthcare. In my opinion, pharmaceutical companies in reality do care if a child contracts Autism from antibiotics or if he dies from

Amoxicillin. Hate to say that, but it's true. They would not be in business if they did not care.

However, if there were a death or tragedy because of some medicine or Amoxicillin, this would be just a margin of error for that deadly circumstance, would be their reply. In some cases, they would just pay out a restitution written off by Uncle Sam. A margin of error that the children of this country do not need and the parents need not suffer. With what I have witnessed over the years in my research, I say it's all about money and volume, not your baby's healthcare that contributes their fortunes.

Sure, I know there is doctors in the country that work from the heart and not for the money. Of course, let us not forget the good people that have completed their studies against Amoxicillin that the medical community refuses to follow. Makes me wonder why the medical communities are not listening to the research that has been done against amoxicillin that is causing major problems against our children. Maybe this group of doctors refuses to listen because they are a large majority, and they have many lobbyists and a full trainload of attorneys by their side. I guess and there is no sanction that says they have to take a different course of action apart from amoxicillin. Maybe that is why I think the medical community refuses to take the advice of these researchers who are against Amoxicillin for infants and children for developmental reasons. Make no mistake; this story is proving beyond any doubt that Amoxicillin has something to do with 1 in 88 children being diagnosed with autism, developmental delay, spectrum disorder. With all the proof I already handed out to you, all you have to do is look at the big picture.

The Amoxicillin Autism Affect in this country must end to stop the production of Autism from going to a figure 1 in 50 children. My grandbaby is living proof of the Amoxicillin Autism Affect, and my research is over compelling to convince me otherwise. Make no mistake this book will be in almost every families home eventually as part of their library, so parents can be reminded about the mistakes I made by allowing my full trust in my grandbaby's four pediatricians 110% for the cure of my baby's illnesses.

It is important to do your studies on your baby's sicknesses and to protect your children from Amoxicillin or any other antibiotic in harm's way to your children. There are other alternatives for your baby; just ask your pediatricians and demand an alternative other than Amoxicillin. They will listen and follow your recommendations but they will not stop administering Amoxicillin to their patients, because it's their #1 drug of choice unless you put your foot down.

Yes, I am an angry grandfather who hates what they've done to my grandbaby and other children over the years. I am hoping that the doctors that hurt my baby will read this book too, so they can see for themselves the truth of the matter. What they did was wrong, and that's the truth of the matter on the subject of Autism. Doctors in this country will ultimately do their research on what I am saying here.

My hope is that they will ultimately stop prescribing Amoxicillin to babies and children with ear infections and other ailments, and start using something else that would stop damaging our babies' immune systems. Please understand, in spite of everything I truly believe that all doctors in this country, truly deep down underneath it all, really care in their hearts about your baby's healthcare. Though some may not realize that indeed they're causing harm to our babies.

All doctors really love children by their code of honor, and the passion they have in their hearts. Of course, I am speaking of a certain group. To me the problem lies in following a protocol routine for prescribing amoxicillin, for just about every type of ailment or sickness that children may have. Doctors listening, and following the recommendations of pharmaceutical company sales representatives. Remember most doctors specialize in the body not in medicine, but they can do a better job in teaching themselves on medicines when working on children's healthcare in the child's lifetime instead of relying on representatives of pharmaceutical companies.

Even if it's just a mild infection that can be cured with another type of medicine less dangerous to the child's system, you as the parent must question the pediatrician about that medicine and do some research on it. The big problem here is not looking at the clear picture on the child's history of all the cycles of Amoxicillin that the pediatricians have prescribed to the child in their care.

The danger lies in causing a build-up of spoors—infectious bacteria in the baby's system as time passes. For me some doctors are too busy looking more toward profit and gain, not realizing that there is more to human life than hitting the top of the mountain when it comes to our baby's and children's healthcare. Eventually if they do not stop the Amoxicillin Autism Affect, parents and child advocates in this country will have to come together to make it happen.

We will even walk to the steps of the White House, and make sure that the President we elected steps up to plate to put a stop to Amoxicillin being the #1 drug for pediatricians on infants and children. When that happens we will see the reduction of Autism Spectrum Disorders and Developmental Delay in this country at a fast rate, and you can rely on that. The big question is: will the medical community finally come to terms with the truth of the matter, that indeed Developmental Delay is caused by excessive Amoxicillin beyond the cycles of danger.

It is and has been compromising our children's systems. Would they truly stop and consider another alternative, to prevent more victims of the Amoxicillin Autism Affect, which is widespread throughout the United States? That is the question! On the other hand, will they just continue excessive regiments of Amoxicillin without any concerns, and ignore this story completely. This is a question that will go unanswered until you the voters, the families, the readers, start complaining about the Amoxicillin Autism Affect, we owe it to our children; we owe it to the families of the 1980s.

I believe the medical community knows that the doctors and institutes mentioned in this book are correct in their findings, but they will not admit to it. They know I speak the truth. The medical community also knows that apart from some doctors and their research of eliminating Amoxicillin as the

#1 drug for children that are harming our babies, we have doctors that have made mistakes in this country involving this antibiotic.

They have changed families' lives forever as well as the future of these children. Still the medical community will not heed unless we do something about it. There is no room for error; every mistake with Amoxicillin that involves human life is one too many, and every mistake should be answered for. The four pediatricians that hurt my grandbaby and altered my baby's way of life forever have gotten away with what they did to my baby.

They got away with this crime, thanks in part to the Department of Health of our government and George Bush who changed the medical malpractice law, making it more than impossible to file a malpractice suit. I will make it a mission in life to make sure this does not happen to another baby in this country by way of publishing this book, and putting it in every mother's hand.

The government knows what they did to my grandbaby, and refuse to answer my call for help, just as they did not answer the call for help with the families of the 1980s. This is another reason why I must tell my grandbaby's story. Part of my mission here is to try to put an end to the acceptance of excessive prescriptions of this drug on children, from parents that refuse to get involved to look at the truth of what is happening here to their child. They do not know any better but to trust their pediatricians on faith.

The world must know the truth. I say this, for all doctors, pediatricians, researchers, pharmaceutical companies who approve Amoxicillin for children's ear infections and any other ailment - the door is open once again on this subject just like in the 1980s. This time the victim in this case is my grandbaby, who made it through the experience of a death trap and staying alive with his will to live, after the Amoxicillin Experiment that almost killed him. Today he is developmentally delayed and Autistic due to 34 cycles of Amoxicillin treatments in nine months. Doctors' experiment gone tremendously wrong! The excuses of environment and genetics when it comes to the subject of Developmental Delay & Autism Spectrum Disorder in my grandbaby's case is not logical, does not make any sense. The truth will prevail this time and a new order on

Amoxicillin must take place in this country. We all know that vaccines have been the topic for many years. I believe that is a subject too difficult to prove, because of lack of evidence on the subject for many years, but when it comes to Amoxicillin the proof is in the pudding. The proof is before you.

However, we must not forget the rare cases that have indeed created skepticism on the subject of vaccines, as we can understand that not every child holds the same anatomy and may not take well to vaccines, but it is very, very, rare on the average. Having your child vaccinated has a wonderful record of accomplishment of saving children's lives from catching polio or measles and other major diseases. It is a blessing we have vaccines. When I was a child growing up, we never saw or heard evidence that the vaccines were harming any child in our time, and we have never witnessed the vast number of children being infected with a disease as we see today with Autism.

Vaccines are a quick process of a few shots that will prevent the worst diseases that can kill a child, and are given to the child in spacious periods. My heart goes out to the "Hannah Poling Case" from Atlanta Georgia, where a judge ruled in her favor, vaccines that were administered to her as a child. Her case, of course, is very rare, something that has never occurred among the millions of cases of Autism in America.

As for the judge - we the people know how often the judges in this country must decide who is right and who is wrong. In this case, the judge is not ruling that vaccines cause autism, but it was the ramification of the case that made the judge decides the way he did. We also see Jenny McCarthy with vaccines, with her account that Evan contracted Autism through the vaccines.

Jenny McCarthy's work with her son to cure him from this disease is admired throughout America. These rare cases must not be ignored, and from there we exercise discretion on when and how we give our children vaccines, and we examine the vaccine very carefully. But it does not prove that vaccines cause autism. Make no mistake; vaccines are important for our children, as they were when we were children. But people have been puzzled for years on how their children are contracting Autism after a normal birth.

It is a sensible solution for parents with an autistic child to look at the vaccines that we give our children for some possible answers, because there's nothing else that we gave our children except the vaccines, while ignoring the antibiotic possibilities. Parents do not consider the antibiotics that we have given our children along the way simply because of trust we have in our pediatricians and our way of thinking. Some parents, including myself, at the time felt that the antibiotics would just be expelled harmlessly from the baby's system.

We thought if the pediatrician is prescribing the amoxicillin to my baby - it has to be safe.

We were wrong in thinking that way, because we have ignored the dangers what Amoxicillin can do to our children's mind and body. The answer has always been right under our noses as I said earlier. We are too busy putting all our trust in pediatricians and doctors in the medical community for the proper healthcare for our children that we just do not bother to stop and look at the big picture.

When we have lower back problems we take painkillers; we never bother to read on the side effects or the ingredients of the drug when indeed those painkillers are killers themselves, eating away your body little by little, a day at a time, and this is a perfect example. The subject of medicine and antibiotics has been the #1 concern with Autism for over 100 years, where the infant and child have had lengthy amounts of consumption of the drug into the baby's system since the early 1900s, when they discovered Autism.

Throughout the years they have added a high number of cycles of antibiotics that will affect the immune system, and the intestinal tract that eventually will cause dangerous levels for the child, something that has been foretold by some doctors but have been ignored by the medical community. Back in the 1980s there were many families who felt that the autism came from the Amoxicillin antibiotics that were administered to their children on excessive treatments. All the families had proof of action; they watched their babies grow along the way while feeding them Amoxicillin for every ear and other infection. That is how they knew it was the antibiotic that caused the change in their child's development along the way. I am sure some of you fine respectable doctors remember that time of 1980s. The more cycles of antibiotic you put in the baby's system, the more chances of infectious bacteria being developed within the baby's system, aside from the growth of bacteria that is already in their system.

The time is now, this is the time is for truthfulness to prevail and prevent any more harm reaching our children. Time for pediatricians to be set free from deceitfulness, and tell the truth to the parents on how critical it is for the baby, not to go through too many cycles by-passing the danger level of Amoxicillin and other antibiotics. Pediatricians must tell the parents this, and explain to them what would happen to the baby's development changes.

Step into my courtroom and sit down next to the jury panel—the jurors of families and children in this country that have been ignored. Let us see what their verdict would be on the subject of the century - Autism at 1 in 88 created by the Amoxicillin Autism Affect. Let us start the recovery process for the good of our children and to better the bad medical reputation that our country has around the world when it comes to the safety of our children!

For once, let us take care of our children the right way and spread this demand so the pharmaceutical company that holds that cue ball can change their ground. I said it earlier - you have to ask yourselves - "why was Autism more becoming common among prominent families in its early history and not the poor"? Why were the parents of the 1980 ignored when their children caught after amoxicillin autism affect? Why is my baby today Autistic? As far as I am concerned, the families of the 1980s, and the horrible Amoxicillin blood bath that my grandbaby endured that made him Autism today, and it is they who have answered the autism question - finally! It was the Amoxicillin! Period!

18
OPEN YOUR MIND

It is a fact, when it comes to visiting a doctor or pediatrician: some people tend to fall into an illiterate state of mind because we just do not understand the language, nor medical terminologies. We do know what is wrong with our baby when they get sick, as well as what is good for our baby, because we love our baby very much and we know our baby better than anyone.

However, what we do not know, is what would cure our baby's illness. So we put all our trust in what the doctor has to say, do, and prescribe for our children's illnesses. Of course, there will be questions on our part as parents and patients. Questions on the medications or exam, or experimenting with an antibiotic for some type of infection that our baby may be having. That is as far as it goes with us parents.

Then trust starts to set in, and we follow whatever the pediatricians have to say from that moment on at the doctor's visit. We worry when our baby gets sick and wonder if the medicine prescribed would cure the baby's illness, but that's when trust sets into our hearts and mind about the medicine, and for the pediatrician that is in charge of our baby's healthcare. Of course, the majority of parents would never think of any medicine hurting our baby in any way, because again, we trust these doctors with our children, thinking in our minds that these doctors took an oath to protect our children's health, so we do not hinge ourselves on a negative thought. Today parents ask the doctor - "Will my baby be alright?" The doctor's reply -"Of course, your child will be fine;" and the parent will go about their business without one shred of concern. Then we find the parent returning a few times on follow-ups for the same ailment.

For many families and their babies in this country, things do not turn out fine at all for their children, especially later on in their children's lives. You might say an internal alternating event will form in time within their baby's system in later years. When that occurs, the baby later on in life starts to develop a change that will affect him or her for the rest of their lives. A most complicated change is when the children are diagnosed with Autism and Developmental Delay later on.

Then the parents get puzzled inside, *thinking how can this have happened to my baby and why?* Therefore, they blame themselves, not realizing that it was not their fault at all. Autism that has a wide umbrella of disorders will fall onto the child, and the challenge will be on the parent to identify and pinpoint which disorder their child falls in. Multi-families find their child at 3 to 5 years of age and are confused with their child's Autistic symptoms because of a normal birth. It is the subversive tactics that the medical community and our government uses to convince the families that the reason for their child's autism is environmental. Ultimately, a good percentage of these families agree with the environmental factors that the medical community speaks of; they have run out of possibilities with the other side-talking environment. However, there is a great majority of families with their autistic children that are not convinced with the environmental or the genes, and have been looking for some answers from the medical community but are convinced otherwise.

These families are convinced, too, as I am that the baby's autistic developmental delay and other disorders are a result of something other than environment and genetic explanations. We are convinced that the results of the antibiotic Amoxicillin are on top of the list. We know our children better than anyone and the events that take place in their lives, not the pediatricians.

The sad part is our own government who is supposed to protect our precious babies." Our Children" does not get involved in these matters.

Even if we go with these complaints to our local government agencies in the town we live in, they will brush you away with no concern. Our government refused to hear the cries and screams of mothers and fathers in this country at one time in our history when some parents first learned the truth of their child's autism, and where it came from. And ever since then it has been a subject that our government refuses to accept. When you hear stories like this - 'no one is hearing the cries of parents'; it makes you wonder about your government and the medical professionals. Are they too busy thinking about their money river cash flows? It breaks my heart. The medical community of the 1980s that rejected the idea that Amoxicillin does not cause the Autism disease - "they were wrong" and they know it! To think that our government would believe that people were never going to come to realize the injury and danger that would follow by introducing Amoxicillin for a permanent stay in all clinics of America, it's just mind-boggling. People are more aware now than ever before in their lives of what is in front of them, and what is behind them.

With this new realization, people will be more aware. When it comes to our children, today is a whole new world in which children get violated through profit and gain with no rights, unless family is there to protect them until the law or death do us part. A tougher love is required for a tougher world. Parents know where their child's illness came from. I thank and credit the parents of the past 30 years who singled out Amoxicillin, but have never been respected or recognized until today - with me.

Life continued in the 1980s for these families, and the outcome of that battle was that the government and medical establishment did nothing about the Amoxicillin Autism Affect of that time. Their complaints were buried in a file. Parent's complaints went unanswered; not even a small research was considered by our government health department based upon their complaints. This would have been the right thing to do when it came to our children, and our children of the future, but nothing was ever done. In that time in history parents were just following doctor's orders about treating their children with antibiotics, and in the end, they saw their children's development change and evaluated their children with autism. Now, look at us 30 years later. One can only assume that there was something more happening back then involving our government and the medical professionals. Whatever it was, I am sure it involved money, profits, and greed. Today, over a quarter of a century later, the problem with autism has reached the danger level, and the government and the medical community are expressing to the world that they cannot say for sure why this is happening?

CNN news and talk shows today throughout America are troubled by the increase of Autism. Fact is we would not have such a high number of autism today if the medical community had put a stop to Amoxicillin, especially, when there were parents demanding it thirty years ago. It is time for the world to know what is going on, and how this government has failed our children.

It is time for the truth on why are we seeing so many children infected today and the buck stops here! It is time to listen, is time to act. It is time for parents to notice things they did not notice before around them! Parents must put on their war gear. We must put on our armor to be warriors for our children against pediatricians and doctors who put negative thoughts and information into our heads about what is right for our children's healthcare.

It's time to put our foot down when they want to fill our babies with Amoxicillin, the number one drug that has been in the spotlight for 30 years. This is our new quest. This is your resolution for your children's life. We must win this battle. Do not be afraid to ask the doctor any question involving your child's healthcare and medicines. We must be extra vigilant, be extra annoying, do not be intimidated by facial expressions coming from your doctor after you get extra precise and specific about the antibiotic Amoxicillin being administered to your baby. The only one that knows the dangers when it comes to antibiotics and babies are the doctors themselves. The pharmaceutical companies and pediatricians must take a different approach and stop cutting corners or taking short cuts on our children's healthcare with Amoxicillin.

They must take the time to explain the whole package when they administer Amoxicillin and other antibiotics to our babies. The danger warning signs of the medications including the risk of death must be explained. All doctors must stop prescribing Amoxicillin to children and babies over an ear or throat infection because they know it just does not work in taking the infection away. These doctors have their foolish attitude: if the Amoxicillin does not work the first time try, try, again.

Doctors go over the duration period of the drug in the challenge to cure the infection and prove to the parents that the Amoxicillin works. This makes matters worse for the child's internal organs. How much money is enough for the Doggie Dog Doctors of this day and age that cannot wait until the day is finished, just to see the profits they made for that day or that week. I am sorry if some of doctors are offended with what I am saying, but truth must be told right here, right now! For all parents, your child may be sick with an ear infection or a throat infection right this very moment, or maybe they're not sick at the moment, which is a good thing. But please heed this information. Start your plan of attack by finding out how much of amoxicillin the baby has taken at different times since birth. It would be irresponsible of me not to share the horribly sad events that took place on my grandbaby in the care of four pediatricians over an ear infection.

I hope and pray it never happens to your baby. However, unfortunately, history shows that my baby is only one among the many millions of babies over the years that suffered the same fate, and all these babies will suffer the rest of their lives for their survival. Worst of all, these families have never applied themselves to stop the injustice that was placed upon their babies through Amoxicillin, and, frankly, neither have I. It takes a lot of money to hire a dream team to seek your justice, especially today.

We cannot stop administering vaccines to our children because we would not want to see our baby develop Polio, German measles, Measles, Mumps and Rubella, Diphtheria, Pertussis, Tetanus, etc. However, we can stop Amoxicillin from destroying our babies over a period with the destruction of their immune system. This story and information you are hearing of my grandbaby is all true, unbelievable, and unimaginable. The information is very vital, very important and very sad to say the least.

For some parents, at this very moment, you could be hurting your baby's health and future without ever knowing it. It is later on in the future when parents come to realize the harm that they caused their baby's development. Parents, it is not your fault that you have been giving your baby all these antibiotics that courses major problems to them later on in life. Parents will come to learn the facts of Amoxicillin only if they do their research.

I said earlier; don't wait years until after your baby is diagnosed with developmental delay or autism spectrum disorder, or any other disorders for that matter to realize that you could have prevented this damage. For the parents of the 1980s, whose children turned autistic after the Amoxicillin Autism Affect experience, I know it's some comfort for you to see the Amoxicillin subject on Autism & Developmental Delay has finally become known once again, and I will not stop thanking you. As for me, I finally open my mind to the reality of what is going on with our children.

Our government health department of the 1980s for our children in this country, and how autism is developing much later after a normal birth. I have finally opened my mind and hopefully the rest of this country will open their minds to this disaster before we see 1 in 50 children being diagnosed with Autism Spectrum Disorders tomorrow. These are the dots that you have to put together, along with an easy equation of looking at the facts of early history, the 1980s, and what is happening today so we can prevent it tomorrow. It all wraps around Amoxicillin since the 1980s and early-history patients. We could not figure out what happened to the early history Autistic patients of rich prominent families, only to assume what really happened by our logic today since the 1980s.

19
THE MALPRACTICE

The lawmakers of this country, lobbyists, governors, senators, pharmaceutical companies, and the President all have children just like us. Their main concern for their children is safety, education, and government. I feel sometimes as though they look down at us like if we are nothing—we're beings that they can control, and taxpayers paying their salaries.

So how can we as a people get anything done for our children's safety when it comes to negligent doctors in this country who are harming and hurting our children? They do not come to our rescue. How can we as a people change a law that our ex-governor left behind, destroying the legal foundation that we had left to get justice for our children whenever a doctor crosses the line in his profession?

How can it be that we elected a governor that has done the ultimate against our children's security, by taking away the only law that would prevent doctors from continuing to destroy our children's systems and changing God's purpose for our child's development. That is what happened in my case. This country has given away billions of dollars to other countries, and what do we get? Higher taxes to cover the bill, and no respect for the American people by changing laws that keeps our people in turmoil, and leaders untroubled by the nation's turmoil involving our children and the hardworking taxpayer. Our children are growing up with disorders and no justice to stop the reckless use of Amoxicillin and other medicines. These children will come to learn how and why they are Autistic. They will all learn about Amoxicillin from their parents.

These children, running into the millions, will run this country in the future. By then I guess they will be the ones to stop any drug that brings harm to the children of America. I guess it has to take an Autistic congressional representative, or an Autistic governor to put a stop to the creation of Autism in this country by rearranging laws that go against the children and people of America. I see a vision that in the future, 30 years from now, we will see an Autistic President. There may be an Autistic majority rule in this country to accept the unexpected visitors with open arms.

The population against Autism will rule this country. I am not saying that would be a bad thing because the way this country is going now it will be a good change in the future. How can men and women who run this country, run it for their own benefit and leave us on the sideline? They are looking down at our children as if they are nothing to be concerned about, because the government has passed laws that go against the security of children. Is it just going to get worse? The New Medical Malpractice Reform Act is to benefit the doctors, insurance companies, lobbyists, hospitals going against our children and victims of malpractice in this country. This law has finished destroying many families, and contributing to more problems in their lives. We Americans know the power to do the right thing for the people takes a President who cares for the people; it was our mistake to elect the wrong person in office with promises of a hypocritical nature. Nevertheless, we learn from our mistakes. Ever since the 2003 Medical Malpractice Tort Act came into law, a number of incredible and horrible stories have emerged.

Some of the first ones to have suffered were the existing malpractice cases already in litigation, or the victims who were just about to file a case against crazy doctors. It was very impressive to hear a judge speak against this new malpractice law on April 27, 2004. Circuit Court Judge Marlene Alva issued an order saying that the new law is unconstitutional, because it retroactively took away vested rights of patients who were already injured by malpractice before the date the new legislation was enacted.

There are horrible stories out there of doctors feeling free to make any mistakes they chose by accident that can hurt, harm, or cripple a child. They can easily get away with it because the caps they put on malpractice will not go far enough to hire an attorney. It is clear that the ex-governor could not unilaterally take away fundamental rights granted by the Constitution, but to take away a child's civil rights to file a law suit against a negligent doctor for misconduct and malpractice, was inhuman to say the least.

It only shows that our children are just little people not to be concerned about. Nonetheless, stories like these cases are appearing all over the United States until this day, more horrible than you imagine. This law is to protect the rich doctors and hospitals alike and to keep the lower minority at its peak. It's a controlling factor of power over the victims of malpractice. The answer lies in the people coming together to abolish this law. We must fight back at this law for the many lives that have been ruined.

You people must come together with the right lawmakers to put this law back into its perspective - away from destroying and hurting lives and causing victimization upon our children and ourselves. We must push this demand upon the new President, this must be done! Alternatively, one day we will see "anarchy" in this country because businesses and people are starting to do business overseas, even going overseas for quality healthcare.

This government used to have quality for their children and families; we even used to export quality merchandise to neighboring countries. It seems that quality and exports have turned to liquidation and imports in this government for the past 30 years, just as they have been dissolving the quality healthcare of our children for the past 30 years through Amoxicillin. Now with this Malpractice Tort Act, it seems they are attacking our inner countries precious commodity by dissolving the civil rights of our children and our people: the right to sue for malpractice against those that harms our children and those that harm our people. If you think about it for a moment this government is destroying themselves, and in the end who will this government turn to for help if the people won't bother lending our government a hand for all their terrible acts upon our own people and our children? Some people say that in the future we will see a second civil war in this country—only it will not be for race but for justice.

Can you blame them for thinking that way? Slowly this country is dissolving. I may not be here for the final hour, but the multitude of Autistic babies and children will be here. I wonder how society will be in the future in regard to our government, and I wonder how our government will be with our society? The makers of the New Malpractice Tort Reform Act is a sure sign that things are just getting worse for the future and not any better.

This is what I pick up among our people because this is a law that goes against what is right for our children and our people, the voters, the families, the malpractice victims. People are very upset with this new change in law that goes against what is right, and embraces what is wrong with this country. A man created this new law and his family morals, a man whom I've never met but just felt his wrath of misery and destruction upon my baby for what these pediatricians did to him.

They created the Amoxicillin Autism Affect inside my baby, and destroyed my family as well as a great many families in this country. The victims are suffering in the hands of malpractice negligence, doctors, hospitals, and health clinics and are at the mercy of the ex-President's Malpractice Reform Act that has affected and continue to affects legal action against gross negligence in this country. The question is why this was done to God's children?

At a time when there are so much complaints on file about quality health care and bad medicine that are, and have been injuring our children for years. I have to assume so many reasons why? How much money was donated to the party from the association of doctors for this new law? Forgive me for being so blunt, but all you have to do is put yourself on the outside looking in, like we simple Americans do. Because of this government's ignorance we will continue to see the growth of the Amoxicillin Autism Affect until the time limit is up.

You can truly see how great government is in not caring for our children that have been infected with the Amoxicillin Autism Affect in preventing their family's justice, from doctors that have destroyed the lives of these children.

This new reform malpractice act is hurting everybody, not only the victims of malpractice, but also the innocent doctors, the good doctors who have never been charged with medical negligence, the ones that care for your health. Some doctors premiums have gone up due to the new reform, and for some even higher. All over this nation, the Medical Malpractice Reform Act that puts a cap on damages has changed rules due to negligence. This is causing great difficulty in getting an attorney to defend the victims of medical malpractice cases. I believe in my heart that because of the new law doctors in this country are willing to take chances on experimenting with their patents with new ideas they create to see if they have a new discovery, like the Amoxicillin Experiment they performed on my grandbaby.

If their new idea does not work and they hurt the baby, they know they can get away with it, because they know that the victim cannot find an attorney to cover all major expenses of the case, and the award being capped will not bring enough money for the attorney and the victim in damages. A destruction of a different kind is occurring in this country Mr. Ex-President, and yes, you have topped the list of Destruction of a Special kind, and yes, you have conquered "the power of control."

As in my case, my little Christopher today has been diagnosed with Autism Spectrum Disorder and is developmentally delayed because of an experiment that went bad from his pediatricians. Of course, your malpractice reform act is able to protect these crazy doctors from gross negligence. Now and forevermore, you cannot sue a doctor for his negligence unless you can prove that the negligence will affect the patient's life later on, even if his negligence almost kills the patient. It may be a negligence that would be easy to prove, but you also have to prove permanent damage later on in life.

It takes the two together in order to sue, and that my, friend, becomes very difficult. Before, you could have filed a lawsuit for the negligence alone - but now, you have to prove both, and good luck finding an attorney. In addition, even if the doctor's negligence may cause harm to the victim later on in life that you may know of, that "later on in life" better hit less than two years, because the statute of limitations only goes on for two years in which you can sue the doctors.

However, in some cases the statute can extend through seven years, depending on certain circumstances. Whether you believe it or not, this is really happening. Our new President is the only one that can change these laws, to add new ones that protect victims against malpractice—laws that are designed to slow down or stop malpractice lawsuits. Victims like my grandbaby will never see his justice because of this alteration in the law. Doctors will continue to experiment with their theories on their patients and continue to get away with harming our children's health for their profit and gain.

I guess this is just another way of killing Americans and causing great harm to our children in the home front, through the medical field and antibiotics that will bring them money. For the rest of our lives most Americans with medical malpractice negligence cases involving antibiotics, and procedures within, will live in misery and will go through this dilemma without seeking justice. I pray every day that God takes his vengeance for his children, and the good people of America. That is all we have left against this massive power that this country has over our children's healthcare. My quest is to stop the misuse of Amoxicillin given to our children, stop Amoxicillin altogether and supply a better option. Eventually it will happen. Someday we will see every child in America taking another antibiotic for all ear or throat infections instead of Amoxicillin, and every child will have healthcare insurance.

For a baby to receive developmental delay and autism spectrum disorder due to the overuse of an antibiotic, it's criminal. If a doctor can do to a baby whatever he wants in the name of guess work profit and gain, and because regulations allows them to, what does this say about our healthcare administration in this country? What does this say about what is happening in this country with our pediatricians and our sick children? What does this say about us for letting it happen to our children?

The Amoxicillin Autism Affect is real and is here to Stay, unless you Mr. President step up to the plate to take out Amoxicillin from every pediatrician's office in America. Fine, if they want to keep it for Adults, but on babies and children it has been devastating.

20
AVOID THE AAA

The US where greed has taken over, and our children and families lives represent just a number to many. Where money talks first and the doctors concerns over your child have a price tag that if you have no money or insurance they will draw you a map, and tell you to make a right turn and go straight ahead for ten miles to nowhere. In reality, with no money or insurance you cannot have the doctor of your choice.

When you take your children to a clinic because they are sick, for whatever the reason may be, pediatricians will make sure that you return to them for medical services, which is the only way they can continue the money train, why? Because your baby has insurance. Even if it's something minor for which you really do not have to return, they will still insist.

Of course, this is good practice to make sure your baby is doing fine. However, when your child is sick with an ear infection or throat infection sore throat, and you find yourselves on Amoxicillin and see yourselves returning to that clinic for over one month, something is very wrong and a red flag should have popped up. If the Amoxicillin did not take away your child's ear infection the very first visit, 7 to 10 days, and you find yourself returning to the clinic more than once, this is a sure sign to stop and think! If the Amoxicillin did not work the first time, what makes you think that it will work the second and third visits? Because the pediatrician is telling you so, "Forget About it!"

Avoid the AAA! Avoid the Amoxicillin Autism Affect! If you allow that, you are heading your baby on the road to AAA. You must not allow your pediatrician to continue giving your baby cycles of Amoxicillin continuing from your first visit to the clinic until your child's ear infection "goes away."

Something is wrong. If it did not work the first time - that's It! Ask your doctor for another option. I cannot tell you what medicine your child needs, but they can. Money is all pediatricians and medical doctors believe in; by making you return to that clinic as much as possible fills up their purse. Whatever you do - do your research on amoxicillin. Your child's healthcare is very important to all doctors, but you have to be on top of your child's healthcare before your doctor.

Have your doctor stay in the examination room a little longer and ask more questions about the medicines your baby has been taking in prior history. Doctors have a tendency to examine the child for less than 10 minutes, says a few words and leave to take the next money ride. No! Keep him in the examining room and have him tell you about the medicines he is prescribing to your baby, all the dangers involved and if the medicine does not work in the first cycle, 7 to 10 days what then? You cannot put all your trust in your pediatrician. I know that may sound a little cold, but it's true. Today we have all kinds of health insurance companies: Medicaid, Medicare, Blue Cross & Blue Shield, and company insurance that pay the bill—the list goes on and on, and that is all they care about. Today we live in a greedy society starting with the fortunate ones and working your way down to doctors. Nothing will change in a doctor's mind and heart about the true meaning of healthcare compared to our doctors in past history who had love and compassion, understanding and who took their oath seriously.

That oath just does not exist anymore. That is why we must be vigilant and in control of our doctor's decisions on our children's healthcare. We must educate ourselves the hard way, be ready to strike the doctor down with his own laws, if it ever comes to that. We must treat these doctors as they treat us, and not be afraid of how they may think; they know our concern may draw questions. You must protect your babies and children at all cost, no matter what happens, and always remember that some of these doctors are not truly honest with you.

For them greed is a good thing, and their job is to make as much money as they can make from your baby's insurance. As for you, do not give in to these doctors' hypercritical smile, and hypercritical concerns. If you show them that you are not a stupid person, they will pretend to see right through you, and be afraid of making a deadly mistake if you treat them with a strong character over the healthcare of your children.

No more Mr. Nice Parent with your guard down. Your pediatrician throws you with a smile. Then you demand to have honest answers as to why your baby's condition is the way it is, and what harm could come to your baby over Amoxicillin? No more lies! No more lies! Since the early 1900s doctors have tried to put their fingers and knowledge on this dreadful illness of Developmental Delay and Autism Spectrum Disorder. Back then, we were dealing with a more honest circle of doctors and physicians in our society of medical professionals.

For me, during the past 60 years, the control of today's doctors has consisted of nothing but lying to the parents. Oh, there is no doubt that there are some doctors who are truly honest and have a pure heart of concern for patients and our children in today's society, but the numbers of dishonest doctors today are overwhelmingly high. I believe for many years now pediatricians, pediatric neurologists, physician's assistants, surgeons, etc, etc, have lied to us when it came down to the subject of amoxicillin and Autism.

The most popular lie of choice started back in the 1970s and the 1980s until this day, when this country allowed hard drugs to hit our streets for profit and greed, because for sure our own government knew about the street drugs. Today when you ask a pediatrician why your baby has Autism - the first reply would be, "genetic or environmental" or "has anyone used drugs in your family in the past?" These excuses were the gold mine to push the parents from the truth of the matter, and the truth is that your child was born normally but after 3 or 4 years you landed in the clinic with Autism

- Why? You want answers, not assumptions. I have done my research and found that taking street drugs does not mean that your child will develop Autism or Developmental Delay or Autism Spectrum Disorder. There are literally hundreds of thousands of babies that have been born normal, with their professional parents having a drug problem. Their children turned out normal with top professional jobs leading to the White House.

Governors, movie stars, lawyers, presidents, police officers, college professors, doctors, nurses, you name the profession - there are literally millions of professional people who have taken street drugs in their lifetime and none of them - and very few of them have children with Developmental Delay or Autism Spectrum Disorder. If street drugs were a leading cause of ASD, then half the world today would be autistic, and practically every member of Congress in America would have children with Autism today.

Of cause, I do not excuse taking drugs. They have been annihilating our country for years, thanks to our weak government on the subject, not to mention the big drug scandal in our history involving third world country and our government that put all those drugs on our streets. Doctors should start talking the truth and asking the right questions, like "Has the child been on any long term antibiotics?" instead of using the drug question.

On the other hand, has the child been eating and putting things in his mouth, and if so, what things? What kind of foods does the child eat? Let us do some lab testing for mercury or any other type of bacteria your baby may have; but they won't ask these questions or do these tastings until it gets more serious for your child. They know that, apart from the good bacteria the baby has in his system, the baby could have had infectious bacteria building inside from all the Amoxicillin they have been giving your baby. These are the questions and concerns parents expect from doctor visits, not a quick flash of the pen and "continue the antibiotics."

However, they will not do that because they have their reasons for not caring to handle the problem correctly and quickly. Unless you are like me and others out there who demand to get the right answers one way or another by proper testing, researching their assessments on the child. Instead they throw the guilt trip at you, so you, the parents of the child, can feel somehow, someway the cause of the problem.—which it originated from you or your family. Thus, they start to point fingers at the parent.

One of the worst replies you would get from your pediatricians and the most popular is that they will tell you not to worry now because it's just too soon to look for any answers.

They will say that your baby is still too young, "let us wait until he is 4 or 5 years of age, and then we will see how he is doing and we will go from there." However, by that time it will be too late for your child to experience any type of recovery. The doctor states those excuses to parents that feel the Autism came from the Amoxicillin. Doctors throwing some hope that maybe the baby will snap out of his illness in years to come. Moreover, of course they will make sure for you to come back on many follow-up appointments. I truly believe that they know by all the antibiotics that they have given your baby, it will cause many different difficulties along the way, and you will be back to their clinic later on. Moreover, you can take that to the bank because it's true! After the Amoxicillin Autism Affect starts to kick in from all the excessive antibiotics passing the duration period, they know you will be back.

I said it earlier in this book that Amoxicillin has a duration period that the antibiotic calls for, especially on infants, babies and children, but sad to say that the Amoxicillin really does not work. Going over the recommended period of the antibiotic will cause breathing problems, coughing, fevers, and diarrhea, side effects from the antibiotic. You will continue to bring your baby back to the clinic for all these occurrences on your baby.

In addition, through it all, they will convince you that your baby has caught that breathing problem in the daycare or that horrible coughing from another child, or those fevers from a change of weather, or that diarrhea from his diet. Making you stay blind to the truth of the matter, they put all the blame on you when indeed it's all coming from all the antibiotics that these pediatricians are feeding into your baby's system, tampering with your baby's immune system. They look at the parents as if it is their fault. Doctors know about the immune system, they have studied medicine as part of their qualifications. If there is one thing that history has shown us about Autism, it's that they could not even assume where and how the disease came into existence, only that it attacked families of stature. Back in the early 1900s we did not have the street drugs of the 70s or 80s as they have tried to put the two together in recent years. They did, however, have doctors that prescribed medicine that has been created through experimenting on human subjects, and used through the 18th and 19th centuries with improvements in the mid-20th century where many of the patients turned autistic.

The bad part of Autism is that the parent always takes the blame until this day. Actually, it is the parent feeding all the medicines and antibiotics to their babies with the doctor's orders, which makes them innocent for hurting their baby's immune system. The parents have put their entire trust on the hands of these doctors who are supposed to care for these children, and it is they that should be at fault for the baby's condition - not the parent!

We are not knowledgeable in the medical department, which is what the doctors are for, to educate us. So do not feel guilty, stay strong and vigilant, you are not to blame for giving your baby Amoxicillin or any other type of antibiotic that is harming your child, but you have to ask yourselves - when is it enough for your child? When do you finally stop? Now that you do know what is going on with Amoxicillin, you can start taking measures for the next time your baby gets sick. You have a sit down with your pediatrician on your next visit and ask her about Amoxicillin, and what are the dangers to your baby's immune system and other organs being affected by it for months and years to come. You go ahead and ask your pediatrician those questions and ask her about other options that will not hurt the baby. Even if it costs more money, you are willing to pay it! You tell her about my book. The big deal here is that you want to try to avoid any possible developmental delay for your baby as time passes. Amoxicillin is one drug that has been in the spotlight for years, you just did not know it; but now you do. I do not want what happened to my baby, to happen to yours. You know what to do! So do it!

21
AUTISM CRIES FOR HELP

Remember a time when war was meant for a peaceful solution and in the end, we shook hands, and continued our lives, living with morals and respecting our fellow man Today wars are meant for power and control over the people and the land. Who are the people that are in control? If you look hard enough, it really is you the parents, the blue-collar worker, the laborer, the meek, the mild, the poor and the innocent. We, the People.

Life has changed for the worse for millions of Americans due to the changes made by governors, senators, Presidents, and our democratic leaders of this country. The men and women who make our laws today should be compared to our founding fathers, who cry down on this country for justice and fairness for the people for thousands of years. A cry so loud that we the little people can hear it every day of the week.

However, for the government and the powerful, these people do not hear anything, not even our cries for help and fairness. We the people have let these unfair laws of this land govern and rule our lives. Now we've reached a point of disaster with our children's healthcare designed to keep the child as part of their purse, whatever it takes. We victims are in pain and craving for help; we can hear the cries of our people, but our government does not. We are programmed only to believe what they tell us to believe, and what we want to hear, so they can be elected into office for their purpose instead of the good will of the people of this country. When will we learn to start putting people in office that care for our people and for our children? Doctors in this country have the power, and the go ahead to feed our children with infectious bacteria through Amoxicillin and other drugs that harm our children forever. Our children are crying for help.

Our governments have laws in place that stop harm towards our children, however, these laws work against our babies, our children, but seem these laws are exempt to doctors in this country. We need people in our government that will protect our children and families of America and stop making Amoxicillin the #1 drug for pediatricians, feeding our babies the recipe for destroying their immune system for years to come.

Where is that poor man in the corner that served this country at war to fight for American freedom, and look where our country put him: in the corner. Let's look for people who know what struggling for their family is all about; these are the true American heroes that we must start electing to run this country; like the ones who have a heart of compassion for all the people in this country. These would be your elected officials to put this country back to its morality, acknowledging what is right and what is wrong for all people, not just for the conservatives and republicans of a country divided. This would be a new commission body for our children's future. This is my vision, a vision that we can make happen, and it will happen eventually. We need people in our government to start caring about our Autistic children, which are growing in high numbers in this country. We must consider that Amoxicillin has caused major problems to our children's immune systems, and to stop the production of the Amoxicillin Autism Affect in this country. One thing this country cannot take away from us is our right to care, and the right to vote. Sure, the politicians keep us down and keep getting richer; but remember one thing, without us they are nothing!

Therefore, we must start teaching our children to stop feeding these politicians with the service they look for from us, especially when they do not fight for our children. I remember a time when the parents of this country had the power to discipline their children, and today a parent will be arrested for doing so. I remember a time when the board of education had the parent's permission to discipline a child, even protect himself or herself from harm's way of a student, but today that has been abolished.

To think that today a teacher has to carry a gun for protection from deranged students is incomprehensible to say the least. I remember a time when we used to say the pledge of allegiance to our American flag of this country in all our schools in this country, and today that has been divided. I remember a time when we used to pray to our Lord thy God of this country, the God of this earth in all of our schools, but today that has been completely abolished.

I remember a time when a doctor used to visit you at your home for the sick, he visited with compassion, especially when it came down to the bill, and if you could not pay it - forget it because God would reward him. That was their attitude. Today a doctor will make sure you pay the bill first before he even says hello to you. When you go to visit him, you have to pay between $50.00 and $250.00 upfront first before he says hello, all in the name of money comes first, and not his concern.

I remember when lawmakers started to change the entire system in this country also in the name of money, power, and control, and to each his own was their philosophy. That was our downfall: <u>To-Each-His-Own</u> and goodbye to everybody else. We took freedom of speech out of context and destroyed it. Today our country is a mess; we disrespect each other and our morals have become non-existent in this country. Today in this country, "Greed" is good for millions of Americans.

It's a completely new crazy way of life in America where if you do not have money - you are nothing and nobody cares! The only way to get by is to fight fire with fire. It's a crazy system so you have to be crazy in order to get by, or play the game, or become a brown nose to your boss, kiss someone's butt, or pay your way through if you have the cash. For the rich, donating money to your Republican Party or to your Democratic Party in order to get a law passed, and later to rule in your favor, and don't worry about the poor because the government has created agencies of different kinds to finish them off, one by one, and to keep them in the palm of agency control. The government is in control of your every move; you are just a television set to them if you are not rich, and they turn you off and on. This is our America today. In addition, speaking of agencies—besides the many crazy ones in existence today— let us pull one out of the hat: The Child Protective Services. Adoption is not what it used to be.

Years ago, it was laid out in a proper format; the parent knew what was best for her child in the essence of raising the child in the proper way. Back then, it was an agency that gave great care and research, with whom a child was to be placed, it, was all-good, and it worked. Today the Child Protective Service is a sad and disturbing crime, and is not a joke. Our government and lawmakers could not care less about The Child Protective Service agency because their children are safe.

Our 2009 Child Protective Services has not changed in the past twenty-five years of major crime and destruction. They are devastating and destroying hundreds of thousands of families here in America. (Do Your Research) The CPS leave behind a record of accomplishment: broken hearts, broken dreams, and childhood destruction. One particular kind of destruction - the rape cases that you cannot imagine. How can it be? Our Government Republicans and Democratic alike, rather than helping our families the godly way, and the righteous way, are ignoring the family. Local governments have used unconstitutional laws in our Juvenile Courts to rip children away from their loving parents. They break our God-given natural parent's family relations, and adopt children of the grieving out to others who profit financially with large monthly adoption subsidy payments. The Child Protective Services agency even has a list of children that they cannot even find, that they have placed in the care of others. It's a long list into the hundreds each year… My heart goes out to all these children in the hands of the CPS.

Moreover, how about the grandparents in this country who decide to rear their grandchildren, because their children are unable to rear their kids. The grandparents are suffering because the government refuses to help them, or even recognize their needs because they have no rights to bear in handling their grandchild. Of course this ignorance goes on because of the government rules and policies that go against the grandparents of this country when it comes to raising a grandchild for a proper and decent life, so it's no wonder that they did not help me with what they did to my grandson's Amoxicillin Autism Affect.

The government would rather take your grandchildren away from you, and throw them into the crazy system with child protective services they have in this country, than to help stop the production of Autism. This is our America the beautiful today - from America with love for the children. It is a cold country when it comes to our children's survival. Autism to our government is all about money and politics with this government un-concerned to evaluate possible misuse of Amoxicillin with doctors in this country.

For me, all I can see is that it's too late to change the commission body that runs this country, because of their greed, power, wealth, and control over the people. However, it's not too late to change the future of this country by raising our children to follow a different path than the path that we followed for the past 30 years blindsided and programmed, that we allowed the Amoxicillin Autism Affect to reach and harm our children.

It's not too late to change this government's way of thinking regarding the security of our children. Bear focus on our ancestors who built this country with their morals and respect for humanity, and the caring they gave our children in this country. It will be a true blessing knowing that before we die - we set forth a new and better way of life for the children in this country and their future. Teach our children never to forget and to keep those powerful words - God Bless America and God Bless Our Children!

22
THE AUTISM RESCUE

As you finish reading this incredible story of why and how my grandbaby contracted the Amoxicillin Autism Affect, there should be no doubt in your minds that indeed my baby's developmental delay and autism spectrum disorder came from the 34 cycles of Amoxicillin given to my baby in a nine-month period, which is unbelievable. I showed you evidence to the fact in this book with studies, and the information in this chapter may serve as well.

We must not forget that some researchers and their study in this country and abroad have substantiated that if you give your baby 20 cycles of antibiotic in the child's lifetime from birth to twelve years of age, he will develop Developmental Delay and Autism Spectrum Disorder. If indeed you give your baby this amount of Amoxicillin, its lethal and deadly, and your baby may very well die.

My baby received 34 cycles in 9 months and lived for me to tell the story. I pray to God every day for my baby's survival, and thank him for giving me the strength and knowledge to tell his story and, hopefully, save millions of children from this controlled operation that has been damaging and killing our children for over 30 years. If your baby is born with a weak immune system, giving your baby fewer cycles than 20 cycles of Amoxicillin, cutting it down to 5 or 10 cycles of Amoxicillin is still worthy of concern. With a weak immune system, chances are that they will still develop a milder form of Autism

Spectrum Disorder and other Disorders. I do not think your pediatrician will ever in a million years tell you that, maybe because they do not know that, or maybe they're too busy. Some of these doctors do not know because they do not follow other doctor's research that may interfere with children's lifestyles.

Since the 1980s with the introduction of Amoxicillin until this present day, we have seen the growth of autism spectrum disorder and developmental delay, making its mark today in 1 in 88 children being diagnosed with Autism. A Record Breaker! Families for years have been misdiagnosed on their child's development, because some doctors just do not care to say early testing would be key.

Families did not know about the Amoxicillin record of accomplishment—the major affects on children, even death, because their children's doctors refused to share all the dangers of Amoxicillin in the name of protecting their #1 drug. Families were not told about the repercussions of giving their children so many cycles of Amoxicillin, and what can happen to the child's immune system. Families brought their children to their baby's pediatrician with a respiratory or ear infection, and by the time the ear infection started to feel somewhat better, that baby would have absorbed too much amoxicillin, starting the process of compromising the baby's immune system to the finish line. This kicked off the process of the Amoxicillin Autism Affect that will eventually kick in. After reading this book, you should know by now not to allow your pediatrician to give your baby Amoxicillin for an ear infection or any minor ailment for that matter. They have other antibiotics that work in 3 to 5 days, and are less dangerous for the baby's system. There are medications or procedures that will not harm the baby's immune system in a timely manner, like what is happening today.

23
A LAW TO REMEMBER

For some there is no financial wall standing in their way in filing a malpractice lawsuit, and for others who are not so fortunate you cannot file that lawsuit against these doctors. The new law protects them by way of – putting a set number amount of what the victim in the case will receive, and its too low for an attorney to take your case. The attacks upon civil trial attorneys represents the ultimate destruction upon our people in America, to hinder the only way we can get some kind of justice for the misconduct, negligence, and malpractice of doctors that are injuring our children.

This attack on our attorneys is not only on them, but also on their clients, including patients victimized by the increasingly shoddy health care provided by some doctors, nurses and hospitals. This attack leaves law firms with no choice but to decline legal representation in cases that indeed have merit, due mainly to these so-called "legal reform" or "tort reform" laws that our ex-President George Bush encouraged. Another wrongdoing for our children with special needs is "money". Shame on Them! Shame, Shame! They should open up charter special schools in every state, paid by tax dollars for our children with Autism, after the harm our medical communities have been doing to our children for 30 years! Yes, we do have some programs, but we do not have enough programs for the vast increase of our autism children, special needs children that were created by our own government laws that allow doctors to do whatever they want with our children.

They're making billions of dollars on our children's disease through health insurance and money out of pocket. To think that this country spends billions of dollars giving it away to other countries and they cannot take care of America's Children with special needs that they created! "Shame on you America, shame on you!" Look at our health care in this country. Is that something to be concerned about? You bet it is! It is time to send out E-mails, right letters to your new President - Let us start making noise for these children.

If you have a story to tell-tell it! Do not be afraid to stand your ground for these children. It is time to get mad, too much wrongdoing is happening to our children and we are lying back too much. This country has the worst kind of arrogance and government officials are enjoying it. The Amoxicillin Autism Affect is real, and it's here to stay. It has been in existence for over 30 years and we have been blindsided, now it's time to wake-up, America! Now you can close this book with this closing prayer, God Bless Your Children Forever, God Bless All Children, May God Bless Little Baby Christopher in Sharing to the World What Needs to Be Done to Stop the Amoxicillin Autism Affect.

IN CLOSING

I know there are those who defend the medical community and our pediatricians with caring hearts. I, too, defend our doctors and pediatricians who save lives and our children. As I said earlier, I just did not get up one day and decide to be an author against the medical community. Forget about it! It's not like that! I respect our medical community and advanced medicine, what I don't respect is when doctors go overboard in a feeding frenzy over excessive Amoxicillin and Augmentin on children, through random treatments creating a long term recipe of destruction for the future of our children creating bacterium's in their system causing the Autism Affect for their future. The parents do not know this is happening to their children! Is it wrong to wake up the medical community about the harm they have been doing to our children for 30 years? Is it wrong to inform parents what they did to my baby and have been doing to other babies? Is it wrong to inform parents about The Amoxicillin Autism Affect?

Please do not waste precious time judging me and this story; children need you to stop this! The truth of The Amoxicillin Autism Affect has been handed out to you. It's not important to me what anyone has to say in disagreement or rebuttal. What is important has been shared and explained to all parents. Parents are the most important people in the world. Parents are the creators from the beginning. I forgive the four pediatricians in my town for what they did to my baby and my family because I believe in God, and, of course, I did not have the funds to higher a dream team. It does not mean that they should not pay restitution if not to me, to God himself. What is important is that you understand that the reason these doctors did what they did is because they were allowed to do it! They followed rules and regulations that allow them to do it. They followed protocol.

Nonetheless, they are crossing over the line of protocol they are wrong tremendously for what they are doing to children, taking advantage of their authority. I am sure these pediatricians have continued to use the same methods on all their children patients, even after knowing what they did to Chris, my grandbaby. Pediatricians today have a one way of thinking when it comes to treating our children, and it's time for us to make it a two way street when it comes to our children. It is time for pediatricians to share the lethal levels of danger in antibiotics that pediatricians prescribe to our children on a random basis. The Medical Community has been hurting children for decades, even causing death to many children.

Every day including this moment children are being diagnosed with autism that has no family history and the children were born normal. The laws involved with the health and welfare of a child in this country must be reconstructed in all levels of government involving the healthcare of a child in this country. These laws should only be labeled to benefit babies and children of this country. These laws should not protect the medical community or even a hospital when harming a baby with Amoxicillin or any drug including death by accident. After reading this book there should be no doubt in anyone's mind what you have to do as a people and as parents, because your children are the most important everything in your life, and your children shouldn't be subject to danger from the medical community that we trust. Amoxicillin is destroying our children's system, thus creating the Amoxicillin Autism Affect. The Amoxicillin Autism Affect is real, and is here to stay, unless you make a difference. This is one challenge that you can take for the first time in your life to do something for these children before you drop and visit our maker. Do not be afraid to take the first step; I took mine, and now it's time for you to take yours. My quest is for every parent to have a copy of this book, pass it on.

God Bless You & God Bless Our Children!

RC GRANDPA

To Jonathan.

I am so proud of you.

Tio - Ralph.